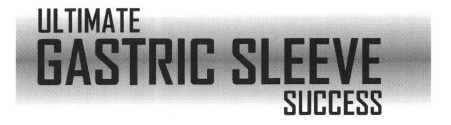

ULTIMATE
GASTRIC SLEEVE
SUCCESS

A Practical Patient Guide

To Help Maximize Your Weight Loss Results

www.ultimategastricsleeve.com

D0041309

DR. DUC C. VUONG

This edition published by HappyStance Publishing.

Print Edition ISBN-13: 978-0615830445
Print Edition ISBN-10: 0615830447

Some information contained in this book might have appeared in other locations, books, publications, videos, or alternative formats by the author.

This book is intended for informational purposes only. This book does not offer medical advice, so nothing in it should be construed as medical advice. You should not act or rely on anything in this book or use it as a substitute for medical advice from a licensed professional. The content of this book may become outdated, especially due to the nature of the topics covered, which are constantly evolving. The information in this book is not guaranteed to be correct, complete, or timely. Nothing in this book creates a doctor/patient relationship between the author and you, the reader. Although the author is a physician, he is most likely not your physician, unless he has seen you in his office as a patient. This book should not be used as a substitute to seeing your own physician.

Cover design, interior formatting, and publishing assistance provided by LOTONtech—http://publishing.lotontech.com.

Acknowledgments

To Hurricane Ike, for teaching me strength and perseverance.

To my patients, for teaching me trust and humility.

To my Dad, for being my inspiration.

To John and Barbara, for believing in me and entrusting me with your daughter.

To Melissa, for teaching me passion and patience.

To Kizzie, our daughter, for teaching me the true meaning of love and joy. May you soon have a little brother.

Contents

Introduction

Much has changed since the publication of my last book, *Ultimate Lap-Band®
Success*, in 2009. After the difficulties following Hurricane Ike, I decided to
leave the struggles of running a private surgical practice in Texas for a
position at a great hospital system in Albuquerque, New Mexico. This move
has given me the opportunity to regroup my thoughts in a nurturing and
caring environment. I can leave the worries of the day-to-day operations of a
medical practice to the hospital and refocus my attention on my true
passion—helping patients improve their overall health by first changing how
they view the world.

Because the comprehensive bariatrics program that I have developed focuses
more on the psychological and emotional struggles of obesity than on the
surgery itself, I have become known as the "Support Surgeon." I consider
support groups to be more important than the actual weight loss surgery
itself. In my clinic, support groups are not optional, and my patients attend
several sessions, even before they have surgery. Following surgery, my
patients abide by the rule that they attend support groups as often as possible,
which typically means weekly. In my opinion, offering a support group
meeting once a month is not frequent enough, because if a patient misses one
month due to a conflict, then that means she will go two months without any
support. I personally lead group meetings in my clinic, sometimes up to three
times per week,, so patients have plenty of opportunities to talk with fellow
patients, meet with me and my staff of weight loss specialists, maintain
motivation, and learn better strategies. Because I interact so frequently with
patients, I have developed some useful insights into the struggles that obese
patients face. And I believe I understand why it's easy to gain weight, but
hard to lose it.

Why It's Easy to Gain Weight, but Hard to Lose It

Human physiology is designed to store energy in the form of fat. We have
natural energy storage areas, such as our liver, muscle, and fat cells. Most
people gain weight slowly over several years, in a stair-step fashion that is
often associated with significant life events, like pregnancy, illness, and

divorce. Graphing it on a diagram, your weight struggles might look something like this:

It is not always a steady increase—usually periods of successful dieting result in bouts of weight loss—but for the most part, it is a slow, gradual, insidious process that happens over many years. Then one day, you wake up, and think, "How did I get this big?" You might get angry or upset. You might blame it on excessive eating during the holidays, your husband's good cooking, or your nagging mother. In reality, however, you most likely gained the weight slowly over many meals, not just one; thousands of food choices, not a few; and hundreds of thousands of daily thoughts, not a smattering of bad thoughts during "stressful" times.

Every time you gained weight, you were eating according to the calories needed at the next weight level. So, if you weighed 130 pounds and gained 10 pounds, you were eating in a way that a 140-pound person would eat, assuming you didn't lose the weight. If you gained five pounds suddenly and then lost it quickly (like around your menstrual cycle), then that increase is more physiological. If you gained 10 pounds during the holidays but failed to lose it, then for the holidays, you ate like the 10-pound-heavier version of yourself. Eventually your body will reset at that state. Some of this is because you adjusted to having that larger portion size. For example, you got used to eating two pork chops instead of one, three pieces of chicken instead of two, and a second (albeit smaller) helping of spaghetti. Once your body becomes accustomed to that larger portion size, you can't seem to go back to the smaller portion size. Two pieces of chicken just don't seem to fill you up anymore. Without that second pork chop, you just don't feel quite satisfied with your dinner. This means that your body's expectations have reset to this new larger portion. More significantly, your mind's expectations have reset. When you gain weight, you have been eating like that heavier version of yourself for a period of time, and then stuck to those new eating habits. But the reverse is not true.

Losing the weight is harder and here is why: you are fighting against your natural physiology of storage. In order to go from 200 pounds to 190 pounds, you have to eat like a 180-pound person—not a 190-pound person—because you are fighting your body's natural tendency to store food. It is like running with a tire tethered around your waist and dragging behind you, or like swimming in a stream against a strong current. You've got to work harder just to get back to the same place!

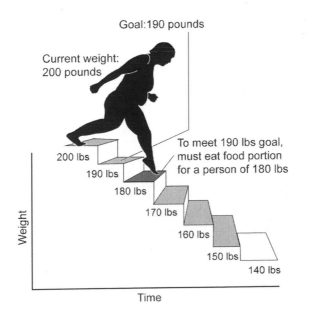

Another way to look at is in terms of food consumption. I think many people can relate to this next illustration. It forms the basis for most diets!

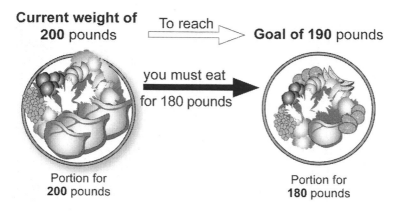

**Current weight of
200 pounds**

To reach

Goal of 190 pounds

you must eat
for 180 pounds

Portion for
200 pounds

Portion for
180 pounds

Please note that the new portion has a lot less meat and many more fruits and vegetables.

Many people talk about our bodies' physiology, but there is more to weight loss than that. There are many currents against which you are swimming in that stream. And one of the most powerful is the psychological current—your own negative thinking. "I can't do this." "It's too hard." "I've failed every diet." I believe these types of thoughts form the most powerful current. Negative thinking is like an anchor around your neck while you are swimming. Everything starts with your psychology, your thoughts. Emotion, how you feel about food, your urges, and your cravings are all tied to your thought patterns, and **negative thought patterns** keep you from reaching your goals of health and happiness.

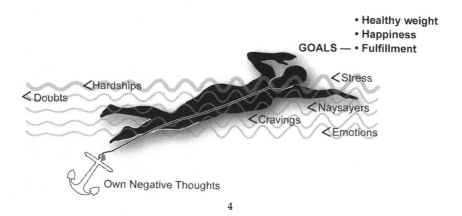

• **Healthy weight**
• **Happiness**
GOALS — • **Fulfillment**

<Stress

<Hardships

<Doubts

<Naysayers

<Cravings

<Emotions

Own Negative Thoughts

What I've come to understand in the past several years is that...

> *In order for you to permanently change your weight, you must change your thoughts!*

For example, you probably looked at the illustration of the plate of food above and thought to yourself, "This drawing doesn't apply to me. There is no way I eat THREE pork chops!" or "I can't possibly eat that much salad" or "I don't like the taste of vegetables" or "One small pork chop will not satisfy my hunger." And all those thoughts would be valid. The illustration is NOT completely accurate. If I had to draw the food plate diagram for the average American, it would look more like this:

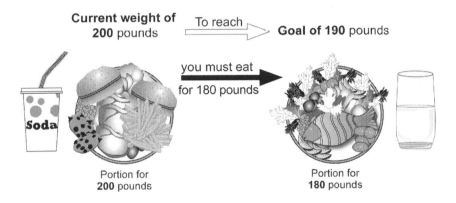

Notice the differences between the first and second food plate diagrams. Most people eat more red meat, junk food, and fast food than they think. They consume a tremendous amount of calories and chemicals from sodas. They eat fewer fruits and vegetables than they'd like to admit. Then when they are on a diet, most Americans don't change the content of what they eat, just the quantity. They do not increase their consumption of fruits and vegetables nearly enough. Most fail to replace the red meats with leaner sources of protein like fish, instead opting for smaller portions of red meat. Lastly, most people do not consume nearly enough water, despite being made of 2/3 water!

"So how can I change my negative thoughts, Dr. V?"

It's simple: Start by changing the words you use to describe yourself. It's not easy to do; it must be practiced everyday. It is simple to get started, but it's easy to get off-track. I will discuss this and other strategies throughout this book.

In this first section, I have included the worksheets and discussion topics that I cover in my key perioperative support groups. I require all of my sleeve patients to attend a minimum of eight weeks of perioperative sessions: three groups before and five groups after their surgeries. This means that patients will come to my office initially for at least eight weeks in a row. I personally lead these sessions, because I believe these topics are critical for sleeve patients' success and happiness. They then must attend monthly maintenance support groups, in which we discuss broader issues like "Body Image" and "Exercise Fitness." This is the minimum requirement, but they are encouraged to come every week. I have some patients who come weekly for a couple of months *prior* to surgery!

Some readers might say, "There is nothing you can teach me, because I already know everything there is to know about dieting. Why should I read this book?" I would like to test that argument right now. Here are some questions that cover information you will learn by reading this book. Try to answer these questions.

1) How many calories are in a gram each of protein, carbohydrate, and fat?
    a. 3, 4, 5
    b. 2, 2, 10
    c. 4, 4, 9
    d. I have no idea what you are asking, Dr. V.

2) Which has the highest amount of protein?
    a. 1 ounce of fish
    b. 1 ounce of chicken
    c. 1 ounce of beef
    d. They all have the same amount of protein.
    e. But what about cheese sticks, Dr. V?

3) Which has more calories?
    a. 100 calorie bag of Oreos
    b. An apple
    c. They are about the same.
    d. If you are standing when you eat, everything has zero calories, right Dr. V?

4) How many calories do you burn from walking?
    a. On average, for every 130 pounds of weight, you burn 100 calories per mile.
    b. Not enough to make up for the junk I just ate for lunch.
    c. Not enough to classify walking as an exercise regimen.
    d. All of the above.

5) The road to weight loss success starts and ends with:
    a. My surgeon
    b. My mom
    c. My spouse
    d. My job
    e. My children
    f. The person in the mirror

You might think you know the correct answers, but what if you're wrong? Are you willing to take that chance and compromise your health? The answers to the above questions are all contained within this easy-to-follow book, so hopefully I have convinced you to keep reading. This book is not just a collection of your typical "dieting tips" with which I'm sure most overweight people are familiar. Instead it is filled with no-nonsense, practical, physical and mental exercises that, if practiced, will keep you motivated until you reach your ultimate goals. Even though I am most likely not your surgeon, you can maximize your learning from this book by actively participating in the content I'm presenting, as if you were in an actual group at my clinic. Follow these steps to get the most out of this book:

- Answer the questions first. Actually write out your answers. **Even if you don't know the answer, take a guess.** You will learn and remember much more if you actively participate in the book. Once you have completed the questions for a section, go ahead and flip to the discussion of that topic.

- Take notes as you read along. I hope to offer you many easy-to-follow tips and strategies for maximizing your success. I intended for this book to be written in! So, make lists of what you will incorporate into your lifestyle now.

- Go back and review your answers after reading the discussion section. This will help emphasize which of your choices need reworking or rethinking.

- Teach these tips to someone else. Better yet, have a friend participate with you. You can compare your answers and what you've learned. In essence, start your own support group, using this book as a basis.

- Revisit the questionnaires every couple of months. You can see which changes you have adopted and then set new goals to keep the momentum going. Then reread the discussion section to see if there are more things you can change to keep you on track to a healthier body (and consequently, healthier mind and soul as well). I've included an appendix of some key concepts I've developed and teach my own patients.

My support groups are topical, so my patients often revisit support groups that focus on their trouble spots, like "Social Eating with the Sleeve." They will come back a month or a year after their first participation in that session to reinforce their knowledge of good sleeve eating habits. So hang on to this book once you've completed it. The first step to fixing those troublesome areas is to think about them. Then keep thinking about them. And then take action. So let's get started!

Understanding Your Gastric Sleeve Surgery

Understanding Your Gastric Sleeve Surgery (Quiz)

I am surprised by how often I meet a patient who doesn't know what type of weight loss surgery she had, much less be able to describe the surgical process. It's easy to understand if the patient's friend or family member is unsure of which procedure was performed, but I'm talking about when the patient herself doesn't know. She can't tell me the type of gastric band that was placed, the type of pouch that was created, or even if the intestines were rerouted. Is this a failure of the patient's memory or a shortcoming of our surgical system? I'm not sure, but it probably has to do with the typical nature of doctor-patient relationships and interactions. Regardless, I never want this to be the case for one of my patients. The following is a quiz that my patients actually work through with me prior to their sleeve surgery.

Draw your stomach.

Draw your gastric sleeve surgery.

What possible complications might you get after surgery? What symptoms might you feel?

What other procedures or tests might you need after your surgery?

What are the recommendations for vitamins after your sleeve surgery?

Why are you having weight loss surgery? What are your specific objectives?

Understanding Your Gastric Sleeve Surgery (Answers)

I am surprised by how often I meet a patient who doesn't know what type of weight loss surgery she had, much less be able to describe the surgical process. It's easy to understand if the patient's friend or family member is unsure of which procedure was performed, but I'm talking about when the patient herself doesn't know. She can't tell me the type of gastric band that was placed, the type of pouch that was created, or even if the intestines were rerouted. Is this a failure of the patient's memory or a shortcoming of our surgical system? I'm not sure, but it probably has to do with the typical nature of doctor-patient relationships and interactions. Regardless, I never want this to be the case for one of my patients. The following is a quiz that my patients actually work through with me prior to their sleeve surgery.

Draw your stomach.

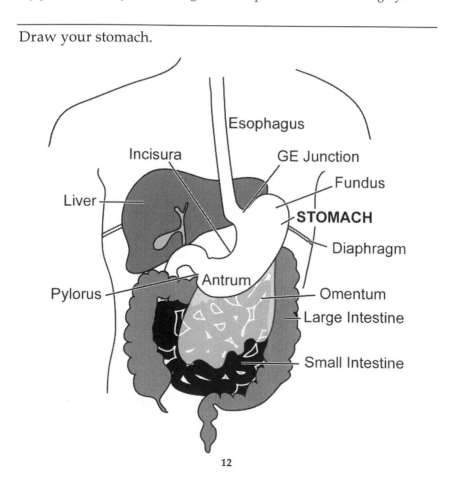

This is a diagram of a normal stomach. Note these anatomic areas:

- *GE Junction:* This stands for the gastroesophageal junction (GEJ), where the esophagus becomes the stomach.
- *Crus (or "crura" in plural form) of the diaphragm:* Your diaphragm is the sheet of muscle that separates your chest (thoracic) cavity from your abdominal cavity. It is a thin muscle, but as it progresses toward the middle of your body, it thickens into a more pronounced muscular pillar called the crus. The opening (hiatus) created by the left and right crura defines where the esophagus, aorta, nerves, and a few other structures come through from your chest into your abdomen.
- *Hiatus:* The opening defined by the left and right crura of the diaphragm.
- *Fundus:* The top portion of your stomach. It has the potential to stretch.
- *Omentum:* The protective sheet of fat that lies over your intestines. We are learning more and more about it every day. We used to think all the omentum did was "shield" our abdominal organs from harm, but now we think that it is an endocrine organ—in other words, it secretes chemical signals to affect biological change in our bodies. The omentum becomes quite fatty with obesity, and scientists now believe this is one of the major causes of the comorbidities associated with being overweight.
- *Greater Curve:* The long curve in your stomach. It is attached to your omentum and lies near the colon.
- *Lesser Curve:* The shorter curve in your stomach. It is thicker and less stretchy than the greater curve.
- *Incisura:* The bend of your lesser curve.
- *Antrum:* The area of the stomach right before your pylorus. It performs a "churning" action that mixes food with stomach juices to speed up digestion.
- *Pylorus:* The muscle at the bottom outlet of your stomach that controls the rate at which partially digested food leaves your stomach and goes into your duodenum.
- *Duodenum:* The first portion of your small intestine that is responsible for a variety of digestive processes.

Draw your gastric sleeve surgery:

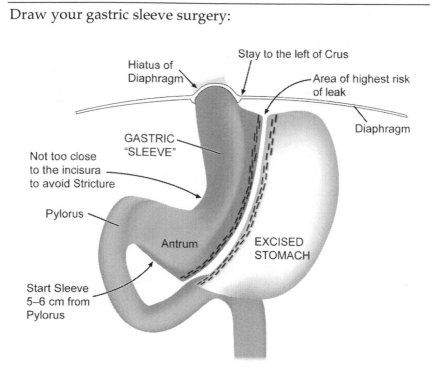

At the time I am writing this book, the techniques for gastric sleeve surgery are still being refined. Surgeons are still trying to determine how large to make the sleeve, how close to the pylorus we should start the sleeve, which device to use to create the staple-line, etc.... In general, surgeons aim to remove about 70 to 80 % of the stomach. Please check with your surgeon to understand the nuances of his or her technique. Here are some guidelines that I learned during training and follow as I perform the surgery:

Stay left of the left crus of the diaphragm to avoid esophageal injury and leaks—Cutting too close to the crus increases the risk of sleeve leaks. We think this is the area of highest internal pressure, which is significantly elevated with postoperative swelling. With too much pressure, a small leak may form. This area is theorized to have poor blood flow, which might affect healing of the stapled tissues. Coming too close to the crus can also injure the esophagus. The esophagus only has two muscle layers, so it is not as tough as the stomach, which has three layers. Esophageal injury can be serious.

Make a small fundal pouch for patient comfort and to avoid stretching—I like to leave a very small fundal pouch at the start of my sleeves, because patients are more comfortable when eating if they have a small pouch where food can sit. Not all surgeons agree with this, so make sure to ask your surgeon his preference before the surgery. There is a fine balance between leaving the right amount of fundus to help patients eat comfortably and leaving too much that can stretch, resulting in weight regain.

Do not leave a redundant fundal pouch—A redundant fundal pouch is very different from the small fundal pouch discussed in the previous bullet point. Sometimes the fundus, especially in tall men, can be hidden from the surgeon's view because it lies near the diaphragm. Unintentionally leaving behind a large fundal pouch as the sleeve is created decreases weight loss success because it can act as a reservoir where extra amounts of food can sit.

Do not get too close to the incisura to avoid stricture—A stricture is a narrowing in the internal opening of your sleeve. Most strictures will occur near the incisura. A stricture may occur if the surgeon gets too close to the "bend" when creating the staple line. Patients might experience food obstruction, nausea, vomiting, and abdominal pain. Correcting the stricture might require endoscopic dilation, stenting, or even additional surgery.

Create the sleeve six centimeters from the pylorus to avoid dumping—I believe patients need some antrum to help them with the digestive process. Starting the sleeve too close to the pylorus might lead to symptoms very similar to the "dumping syndrome" that plagues gastric bypass patients. Dumping syndrome occurs after the ingestion of simple sugars and is characterized by nausea, vomiting, abdominal cramps, and diarrhea. The six-centimeter distance is by no means standardized; some surgeons will start the sleeve at four or five centimeters. I know of a surgeon who starts the sleeve at the pylorus, which in my opinion, is too aggressive.

What possible complications might you get after surgery? What symptoms might you feel?

Now that you have a better understanding of the surgical anatomy and the possible complications of the surgery, the symptoms of those complications should be clearer.

Leak—This is the complication that worries surgeons the most about the gastric sleeve. Like a leak in your kitchen sink drain pipe, a gastric sleeve leak is an opening somewhere along the stapleline that allows gastric juices to flow out from your sleeve into your abdominal cavity. Although patients with the gastric bypass may also experience leaks, those occurring in gastric sleeve patients are more complex because the sleeve is essentially a high pressure tube. Surgeons are still debating the best ways to prevent, repair, and heal gastric sleeve leaks. Most leaks will require a return to the operating room or another procedure to correct them. I have had two patients with leaks, and luckily they both healed relatively quickly. However, I've heard stories from colleagues who have had quite a difficult time healing leaks, which have sometimes required several months of treatment. Take this complication seriously and follow your surgeon's instructions not only after, but also BEFORE surgery.

Stricture—If you experience frequent nausea and/or vomiting while eating, then you should see your surgeon to be evaluated for a possible stricture. A stricture usually presents as "food getting stuck." Think again of the old drain pipe beneath your kitchen sink. Over time, corrosion, grease, and grime will narrow the pipe's opening, eventually causing a clogged drain. Strictures most often occur at the "bend" of the stomach called the incisura, but they can occur anywhere along the staple line. Your surgeon will probably want to do some x-ray studies, like the barium swallow, or perform an endoscopy. The surgeon will especially want to perform such tests if these symptoms persist after he has analyzed your eating patterns and you have adopted any recommended behavioral changes. Treatment of a stricture often requires an endoscopy with balloon dilation. Some surgeons might try putting a temporary stent in the narrowed area, but in some cases, the stricture might require another surgery to correct the problem.

Oddly, some suspected strictures are not true strictures at all. There have been cases where the sleeve bends, kinks, or twists at the incisura in a way that is not visible on any diagnostic study and only becomes apparent when the patient eats. This can be very frustrating for the patient, who is told that all the tests are "normal," and also frustrating for the surgeon, who is trying to help. Ultimately, such a case might require a surgery to look at the sleeve itself, and even then it might not be apparent. At that point, you have to rely on the experience and clinical judgment of your surgeon, which goes back to my point that you had better LOVE your surgeon—so, find a good one!

Dumping—I am starting to hear about a few sleeve patients who develop symptoms very similar to dumping syndrome, namely nausea, vomiting, diarrhea, and crampy abdominal pain after eating. I suspect the condition occurs when the sleeve begins too close to the pylorus, cutting out the grinding function of the antrum and creating too short of a transit time into the small intestine. The number of patients with this problem right now is anecdotal, which means that I hear about such cases at professional meetings or have a few patients with this problem in our separate practices, but no study has yet to be conducted on it.

Sleeve irritation—If you experience pain when eating, you might have irritation of the gastric lining. The sleeve gastrectomy is an acid-inducing procedure, at least initially. If you do not take an antacid (preferably a type of medication called a proton pump inhibitor or PPI), or if you eat or drink foods high in acid, like tomato sauces and coffee, you might irritate the stomach lining. If you continually eat too much or swallow bites that are too big, then that big bolus of food, once lodged, can irritate the lining. So remember to take your PPI, avoid high-acid foods, and most importantly do not overeat!

Ulcer—A lot of times when patients—especially gastric bypass patients—have stomach ulcers, they will actually lose a lot of weight! This is usually because they experience significant pain with eating, due to the inflammation and raw surface of the ulcer. The ulcer can also bleed, causing some patients to become anemic or have dark, black, or tarry looking stools that are particularly foul-smelling. Bleeding ulcers can cause patients to lose a significant amount of blood, which can result in anemia, the condition where the body's amount of hemoglobin, the molecule that carries oxygen to your tissues, is too low. A bleeding ulcer will probably require an endoscopy procedure.

Anemia and Vitamin Deficiencies—Most gastric bypass patients will develop a mild anemia, due to the malabsorption of the nutrients that the body needs to make hemoglobin, such as iron and B12. Bypass patients should always take their supplements and routinely have labwork to check for anemia. This is not such a common problem for gastric sleeve patients; however, if you're not eating foods that are high in iron, like spinach, and continue to eat empty calories, like chips, then you, too, might develop a mild anemia. Even people without any weight loss surgery who do not eat nutritious foods can develop anemia. Overall, most doctors believe that the risk of anemia and nutritional deficiencies should be lower for sleeve patients than for patients with weight loss surgeries where intestinal rerouting is involved.

Weight Regain—Weight regain has two possible causes: 1) a problem with the surgery; or 2) a problem with the patient. If a patient is regaining weight, then as her surgeon, it is my responsibility first to make sure there is nothing wrong with her sleeve. Has the entire sleeve stretched out? Has the fundus (top part of the sleeve) stretched out, creating a big pouch? Is there a stricture or ulcer that is causing my patient to eat soft foods (see the section on Mushy Food Syndrome in the Chapter on The Texture Scale), which are typically high in calories and low in nutrition? Has my patient started taking a medication or supplement that induces weight gain, like steroids or antidepressants? Once I have eliminated a medical or surgical cause, then I turn my attention to a possible patient cause.

Have the old bad habits crept back into her life? Is it stress eating? Boredom? Loneliness? Has she recently gone through a divorce, lost her job, or lost a loved one? Did she have an accident and now can't exercise like she used to, so that the balance of caloric intake and energy expenditure ratio is off kilter? Sometimes patients just need to be reminded, like we all do from time to time, that WE ARE WORTH IT! Don't give away all the hard-fought gains you've made along your weight-loss journey.

What other procedures or tests might you need after your surgery?

Barium Swallow—Most surgeons will perform a simple contrast x-ray study called a barium swallow the day after your sleeve surgery. They might also order it later if they suspect a possible problem with your sleeve. This test is usually performed in the radiology department of a hospital, but some surgeons have a fluoroscopy machine in their offices. You will drink a small amount of a chalky, white liquid that is denser than your tissues. Then, x-rays are taken to see how the fluid travels through your gastrointestinal (GI) tract. The contrast between the barium and the density of your tissues allows the surgeon to see the lining of your esophagus and your sleeve, so he can assess the look of the transition from the esophagus into the sleeve. He can detect a hiatal hernia, strictures, a dilated sleeve, or a retained or stretched pouch. He can also see how the contrast solution empties into the small intestine. This is all very good information, but it has its limitations, too. For example, we only get to see the outline of the GI tract and not the actual tissues. To do this, most surgeons will also recommend a test called an esophagogastroduodenoscopy or EGD for short.

EGD—This is an endoscopy procedure performed by inserting a small soft camera into the patient's mouth when the patient is under mild sedation. Often it is performed for reasons unrelated to bariatric surgery, like abdominal pain, reflux, or stomach ulcers, but it is also very helpful after weight loss surgery. The EGD allows surgeons to visualize your GI lining to check for irritation, ulcers, and bleeding. Not only can we measure how big your sleeve is, we can also see if it has any strictures or kinking. An EGD also gives us the ability to perform any necessary tissue biopsies that can't be done during a barium swallow. We can assess the contraction of the esophagus and pylorus (the muscle that controls the emptying of your stomach), although a barium swallow is better for that. So, you might need both procedures.

Blood Work—At the very least, you should have routine annual blood work. The baseline numbers are important to confirm that any illnesses related to obesity (comorbidities) are improving. Are your blood glucose and hemoglobin A1C coming down? If so, that's an indicator that your diabetes is improving. Are your liver enzymes returning to normal levels, showing that your liver is recovering from the damage of poor dietary choices?

Blood work is also important to make sure you are not developing new problems, like vitamin deficiencies. Deficiencies in vitamin B12, folate, vitamin D, iron, and calcium are common in the bariatric population. They are worse with malabsorption procedures, like gastric bypass or the duodenal switch, but can occur in sleeve patients (Gehrer, 447.) Why is this? Even though you've had a sleeve, you still MUST change what you eat. What you ate previously probably didn't have much nutrition to it. An Oreo is still an Oreo, whether you eat it before surgery, with a sleeve, or after gastric bypass. I LOVE Oreos, but I know they are not good for me, so I don't eat them often.

Most obese people, though large on the outside, are actually malnourished on the inside.

What are the recommendations for vitamins after your sleeve surgery?

I recommend taking a multivitamin that is made specifically for bariatric patients for one year after surgery. You will need the supplements as you learn how to eat again after surgery (Snyder-Marlow, 600.) Learning nutrition takes time; breaking bad habits takes time. Remember, chips are still chips, even after weight loss surgery, and cookies are still cookies. These "foods" have very little nutrition, so you need nutritional support as you begin to change your diet. We know now that a simple multivitamin a day is probably not good enough for weight loss surgery patients, especially for gastric bypass patients. The ones designed for bariatric patients are usually formulated to have higher bioavailability levels. After a year, my goal is for my patients to obtain all the nutrition they need from the real foods they eat. You should not need to live off protein shakes, protein bullets, or anything else that has been pre-packaged for you. Gastric bypass and duodenal switch patients are exceptions, because they physically can no longer absorb as many nutrients from food. But there is no malabsorption with the sleeve, so you should comfortably be able to get enough nutrition from eating fresh foods.

Why are you having weight loss surgery? What are your specific objectives?

Many good (and bad) reasons exist for going through with weight loss surgery. Some patients think, "Boy, have I really gotten THIS bad? Have I REALLY reached the point where I need weight loss surgery just so I can live my day-to-day life?" These patients accepted the need for medicine to control diabetes or blood pressure and assume chronic joint pain is a natural consequence of aging, but when day-to-day life became too difficult, they decided to take action. The realization that they have reached this point can be overwhelming for some patients. That is why it is important to think about this question BEFORE you have surgery; otherwise, the reality of it all might be too much after the surgery.

Here are some examples of good reasons patients have for proceeding with weight loss surgery:

"I need to do it for MY HEALTH."

"My knees (back, body, hips) hurt too much for me to get through the day."

"I'm tired of taking all of these medicines (shots, doctor visits, blood draws, etc...)"

"I'm worried that if the electricity goes out during the night and my CPAP machine stops, I might not wake up the next day."

"I'm sick and tired of being sick and tired."

"I need to do it for ME."

"This person is not the real me. I want to start living like the person I was meant to be."

"I feel like I'm being passed up at work (didn't get a job, promotion, etc...) because of my weight, and therefore, I'm not making the amount of money I need for the life I want to live."

"I want to leave behind a better legacy, including great memories of fun times."

"If life is this hard now, my 'golden years' will just be miserable."

Here are some examples of not-so-good reasons to have surgery:

"I need to do it for OTHERS."

"My kids really want me to have it done."

"My sister (mother, friend, etc...) had the surgery, and it worked for her."

"This will save my marriage."

"My doctor told me I won't live 5 more years if I don't have it done."

"I'm going to lose weight and show all of those people who used to pick on me in high school."

"I got the money in the divorce, and I'm going to show my ex-spouse that he can't tell me what to do with it."

If you have surgery for someone else, you will probably not be successful. Sure, you might lose some weight at first, but if you do not have a high level of commitment to changing your life for yourself, you will likely regain it all. Remember, gastric sleeve surgery is not a diet, and it's not a quick fix. Gastric sleeve surgery is a life long commitment, so you must know as much as you can about it before saying, "Yes. This is right for me."

Preoperative Sleeve Knowledge Test I

Preoperative Sleeve Knowledge Test I (Quiz)

Determine how much you know about the gastric sleeve procedure, so you can be sure you have accurate expectations.

With the gastric sleeve, I will be able to eat:

a) *Anything I want right away.*

b) *All breads and meats.*

c) *About 1100 to 1200 calories a day.*

Immediately after surgery, I will:

a) *Wake up skinny.*

b) *Have some discomfort that should get better gradually.*

c) *Go on a long trip.*

With the sleeve, I can:

a) *Drink all the alcohol I want and expect to lose weight.*

b) *Eat all the ice cream I want and expect to lose weight.*

c) *Have sweets and alcohol (in moderation) and expect to lose weight.*

d) *None of the above.*

I need to start an exercise program.

a) *Before surgery.*

b) *After surgery.*

c) *Never! Exercise is a bad word.*

Write down six super foods.

Preoperative Sleeve Knowledge Test I (Answers)

Determine how much you know about the gastric sleeve procedure, so you can be sure you have accurate expectations.

With the gastric sleeve, I will be able to eat:

a. *Anything I want right away.*

> **False.** There is swelling around your sleeve for a few days or weeks after surgery, meaning that its open channel might only be a few millimeters wide. Patients are often surprised when I show them on their postoperative swallow study the thin line that represents the internal lumen (or open channel) of their sleeve. Sometimes it's only as wide as a pencil tip. It is not possible to predict the amount of swelling that your body will experience or exactly how much pressure is pushing on the staples holding your sleeve together. The gastric sleeve is a high-pressure system, which means that it functions very differently from a gastric band or gastric bypass surgery, so it is very important that you follow your surgeon's postoperative guidelines closely.
>
> I always keep my patients on a high-protein liquid meal-replacement program, like Optifast®, for one week after surgery. This is to prevent any food from getting stuck. If food gets stuck, you will have a lot of pain and possibly vomit. This will put you at risk for developing leaks and other complications. After liquid meals for one week, my patients go to mushy foods for one week. I then transition them quickly to solid foods. I discuss the reasons for this later.

b. *All breads and meats.*

> **False.** Immediately after surgery, you should go on some type of liquid diet. Please follow your surgeon's guidelines. Unfortunately, there is no standardization among surgeons, so don't be surprised if you have to do something your friend didn't, or vice versa. Eventually (about 12-18 months post-surgery), you should be able to eat most foods. During that time, you will increasingly add different foods back into your diet.

The long-term food tolerance is different for every patient. Some patients can eat bread and some can't. Some can eat steak, but not chicken. Some used to be able to eat eggs, but after a sinus infection, they can't. There are no rules about how an individual's body will react. I think this variation probably has more to do with psychological and mechanical eating factors than it does with the sleeve itself. Here are two things I tell my patients that I believe are true for every person.

Bread for the most part has very little nutritional value, but can expand and take up a large amount of space in your sleeve, so try to avoid it.

If you never eat red meat again, you will likely live longer and be healthier.

c. *About 1100 to 1200 calories a day.*

True. Once your sleeve has healed and the swelling has gone down, your caloric intake should hover around 1100 to1200 calories per day. This amount will keep you satisfied and result in safe but dramatic weight loss IF you eat real food and do not take in empty calories. After all, you could consume 1100 calories with just one McDonald's milkshake and almost zero vitamins and minerals to keep you feeling energized.

What is "real food?" Think...Caveman! This is a tip that I learned from Dr. Kevin Prentice from Dallas. He is a chiropractor, but knows a lot about healthy eating. He says to think like a caveman when you are making food choices and eat only what a caveman would quickly recognize as food. A caveman ate fresh meat, fruit, vegetables, and grains. He would recognize a potato, for example, but not a potato chip, so put the potato and not the chips in your shopping cart. Real food is not processed and does not come in shiny packages. It is usually located on the outer edges of supermarkets. Another way to tell if something is real food is if it comes with either no list of ingredients (e.g., an apple) or if you recognize all the ingredients listed on its packaging.

Once my patients have insurance preapproval, I require that they start a 1200-calorie per day diet and lose one pound in one week before they can start their liquid meal-replacement program, which helps prepare their bodies for surgery. If they don't lose that pound, they have the pleasure of repeating that 1200-calorie week. I do this not to punish them, but rather to prove to them that they CAN lose this weight! They don't need any special gimmicks or aids. If they eat 1200 calories of real food, most of them will lose three to five pounds that week (this is after already losing several pounds during their insurance pre-approval period.) This step is important in giving patients a sense of power over their weight-loss journey. If they start regaining weight after surgery, I can remind them that they were successful BEFORE the surgery on 1200 calories, so they can be successful afterwards.

Immediately after surgery, I will:

a.   *Wake up skinny.*

False. We all wish this, but we know it just doesn't work that way. Most of you have struggled for years with your weight, so you can't expect it to evaporate overnight! But I have met more than a few struggling patients at my talks who honestly thought they would wake up and look like supermodel Kate Upton. I have yet to decide if this is a problem with the patient or the program they went through. What do you think? I know that we as surgeons need to do a lot more to prepare our patients BEFORE surgery. This is what my program is all about. I try to empower my patients by encouraging them to understand that their weight loss success is ultimately up to them.

b.   *Have some discomfort that should get better gradually.*

True. The perception of pain is different for every patient, but many studies have shown that pain is significantly less after laparoscopic surgery than after traditional, open surgery. The return to work and normal daily activity is also faster, but this really depends on your occupation. Check first with your surgeon before starting any major activities. On average, most of my patients return to a desk job in 10 to 14 days and to heavy work in four to six weeks. Of course, this timing could be longer if you have a surgical complication. Once patients are discharged from the hospital, they should focus on staying hydrated with water and walking short distances slowly five to six times a day.

28

Patients can also have a referred pain to their shoulders. This is usually due to irritation of the diaphragm during surgery that postoperatively causes pain to be felt in the shoulders. Pain should gradually improve each day, but if it persists longer than normal, it could be a sign of something wrong—so always have your doctor's phone number on speed dial. A fever over 101.5° F, especially when accompanied by chills, is of particular concern. **Do not ignore this combination of pain, high fever, and body chills**.

The most common complaint after sleeve surgery is nausea, but we have good medicines for that. For example, I put a scopolamine patch behind my patient's ear before surgery. Immediate postoperative nausea can be a result of an operation high on the stomach. This occurs in other surgeries, too, not just gastric sleeves. A lot of times, it can be a lingering effect of the anesthetic drugs used to put patients to sleep. Nausea after you are discharged from the hospital is usually caused by drinking too big a swallow too quickly, so go slowly on your liquids. Definitely do not eat anything until cleared by your surgeon!

c.   *Go on a long trip.*

False. Immediately after surgery, travel is not recommended. The number one cause of death in people undergoing weight loss surgery is not the surgery itself, but rather pulmonary embolism. Pulmonary embolism occurs when a blood clot in your leg travels to your lung. To combat this, we give patients a blood thinning shot before surgery and usually again during the hospital stay. If you have a history of blood clots, your surgeon might send you home with daily shots of blood thinning medicine. The most helpful thing you can do to prevent blood clots is to walk.

If patients go on a long trip, like on a plane or in a car, they are at risk of not only developing blood clots in their legs from sitting still too long, but also not even enjoying the trip. Most patients don't know enough about "life after weight loss surgery" to be able to have fun. They might be scared to eat at all and become hungry and anxious; they might fill up on margaritas and become malnourished and ill; or they might be embarrassed to tell anyone they had surgery and feel pressured into eating something solid, which could hurt their staple line. Check with your doctor before you make any long travel plans, and please don't schedule your surgery around the time of a big trip.

If you are leaving the country for surgery or if you live far from the nearest weight loss surgery program, then after your surgery, please remember to stop the car every hour and walk for at least 10 minutes.

With the sleeve, I can:

a. *Drink all the alcohol I want and expect to lose weight.*

False. This is my patients' favorite subject! I know they are tired of hearing me go over this every week, but here we go...1) How many calories per gram of protein? Answer = 4. 2) How many calories per gram of carbohydrate? Answer = also 4. 3) Now, how many calories per gram of fat? Answer = 9! In other words, a chunk of fat has more than twice the calories of a chunk of carbs or protein. If you can't remember the numbers, that's ok. It is the ratio that is important. Another way to look at it is that for the same amount of calories, you could eat more than twice the amount of carbs or protein. Here is the punchline: 4) How many calories per gram of alcohol? Answer = 7! Everybody knows how bad fat is at 9 calories per gram, but many don't realize that alcohol is right below it at 7. There have been many weight loss surgery patients who have lost weight and put it all back on with alcohol. Much of the time, alcohol is consumed along with highly caloric mixers, making a margarita top 600 calories. If you have a problem controlling your alcohol intake, please seek professional help. Get a handle on this before having weight loss surgery; otherwise, weight loss surgery might not work for you.

b. *Eat all the ice cream I want and expect to lose weight.*

False. Despite what Einstein might have thought about compound interest, I think ice cream is the most powerful force in the universe. No weight loss surgery has a chance against it, even gastric bypass. "But what about dumping syndrome?" you ask. Here is the truth: Not all gastric bypass patients get dumping syndrome, and of the ones who do, MOST will lose it after a few years. So, if you have a sweet tooth and are planning on getting a gastric bypass, do not EXPECT the bypass to cure you of your desire for sweets forever.

I enjoy a bowl of ice cream on special occasions, but if a whole tub of ice cream has comforted you in the past, do not fool yourself into thinking that "just a taste" will be ok. That taste will turn into a lot more. And remember, the gastric sleeve works by helping to control your appetite so that you consume fewer calories; it does not erase the high calories in ice cream or other treats. (More about Empty Calories later.)

c. *Have sweets and alcohol (in moderation) and expect to lose weight.*

False. This is the most debated question in my clinic! Here is my stance. If I am ever called to testify about this in court, I will say to the judge, "Judge, I swear I told them never to eat sweets and never to drink alcohol." But the truth is, there will always be special occasions, vacations, and celebrations. This is why I developed the 21 Days Exception, which we will discuss later. A lot of patients tell me, "Dr. Vuong, if I knew what moderation was, then I wouldn't be here to see you for weight loss surgery." There is truth in that for sure! Also, you can't eat ice cream and EXPECT to lose weight. It won't happen, even if the ice cream carton says "Skinny Cow" or "Sugar-Free" on it.

You have to be aware of temptations and acknowledge the choices that you make. If salty chips are your downfall, then don't believe that you can stop with just one, and don't buy a big bag of them to tempt you. Don't allow that ice cream carton or those cookies into your house. If your family complains, remember that if junk food is not good for you, then it's also not good for your family. The types of decisions you will need to make in order to be successful with your sleeve will become clear by understanding yourself through self-exploration and honesty. You can start by defining what "moderation" and "expectation" mean to you.

> *Everything you have in life is a result of the choices you have made, so choose wisely!*

d. *None of the above.*

True. This is the correct answer. I think the difference between "c" and "d" is OFTEN the reason people hit "Weight-loss Plateaus," a concept that we don't believe in at my clinic. In other words, if I had to guess, MOST people who "can't get off the last 20 pounds" or have stopped losing weight for "no apparent reason" would probably answer "c" to this question, and perhaps they need to redefine "moderation" or (even better) cut out all sweets to see the last pounds drop. But I'm sure a few would answer "d" and something else is the culprit. There is always an answer to why you've hit a plateau, whether it is physical, emotional, or psychological.

I believe, however, that unsatisfactory weight loss is probably due more to POOR NUTRITION than anything. We talk way too much about counting calories in this country and not nearly enough about nutrition.

If you have reduced your excess calories to the proper amount and have stopped losing weight, then it is because of WHAT you are eating, not HOW MANY CALORIES you are consuming.

For example, a cookie and an apple both have about 100 calories, but the nutritional content is not even close between the two. A cookie has very little if any nutrition, but an apple has a lot of nutrition. Can you eat five cookies in one sitting? I know I can, though I try not to. Can you eat five apples in one sitting? Maybe, but have you? After one apple, I'm usually done, but that second cookie always calls out to me. Yet a cookie doesn't work for me, my body, and my health, but an apple does.

I need to start an exercise program.

a. *Before surgery.*

True. It is likely that you need to think of "exercise" in a whole new way. Understand that, for most patients, starting an exercise program before surgery just means increasing your activity level. Do not waste your time purchasing expensive exercise equipment or gym memberships! And if you haven't run in 15 years, you will be miserable if you try it immediately. I have too many patients who tried to do the latest "Boot Camp" fad and ended up hurting themselves. They usually pull a muscle in their knee or back. Regarding exercise, I tell my patients,

> *"Any activity you do that causes you to break a single bead of sweat can be considered exercise."*

You can do this by parking further away from where you need to go, walking around the office, using the stairs instead of the elevator, taking out the trash once a day instead of telling your kids to do it, sweeping the porch, raking the yard, etc. **But remember, if you no longer sweat while doing that activity, then it is no longer exercise.** For example, when you weighed 300 pounds and walking once around the block made you sweat—that was exercise. After two weeks, maybe you stopped sweating after one block—then a walk once around the block ceased being exercise. Your body became accustomed to it. So what do you do? KICK IT UP A NOTCH! Walk farther, pump your arms, walk with weights, walk faster and faster and faster, until you eventually start running.

"Physical fitness" is different from "daily activity" and has been shown to extend lifespan and improve overall quality of life. Physical fitness is accomplished by a regular exercise regimen that is done about three times a week and is designed to stimulate your heart rate to a goal target rate. It also includes resistance work with weights. A local gym or college often provides affordable personal trainers who can help design a safe and convenient program for you to improve your physical fitness. Plus, by increasing your level of daily activity, you will also be improving your level of physical fitness, so don't wait. Find something you love that is easy to do, and get started now!

b.   *After surgery.*

False...sort of. Waiting until after surgery is not ideal, but it is better than nothing. You can always start by just implementing the small daily tips listed above and others you may think of. As you lose weight, you will probably feel up to longer stretches of activity at greater intensity. But you've got to keep it up! You must choose to go and do it, not wait until later, or after the party, or when the kids are asleep. If you resist thinking that exercise means going to a gym class or running three miles and think of it instead as manageable bursts of activity, then you don't need to wait until later. You can do it on the way to the party, or with the kids, or right now!

c.   *Never! Exercise is a bad word.*

So very false! Remember how joyous it was to run, jump, roll, climb, dance, and delight in all sorts of movement when you were a kid? You didn't think of it as exercise then, and you certainly didn't think it was awful. In fact, missing recess in the playground was probably a devastating prospect! **Try to think like a kid again and find activities you enjoy.** Even better if they raise your heart rate! You'll probably be able to do more and enjoy moving more as you become healthier. This is an exciting time to rediscover old interests that had you moving around or explore new hobbies, like playing frisbee with your kids or grandkids, or gardening. Once you rethink the concept of exercise, you can develop a more systematic approach.

Write down six super foods.

A lot has been written lately about "Super Foods." Turn on the television, and you will find something on some great "new thing" recently discovered in the Amazon jungle. You will see it talked about on the morning shows or explained neatly by Dr. Oz. There is usually some accompanying headline about "Antioxidants" or "Free Radical Scavenger" or "High in Omega-3 Fatty Acids." Well, let me simplify it for you and name a few. This list is by no means all-inclusive.

Blueberries
Kale
Tomatoes
Beans
Soybean products like tofu
Whole grains like quinoa
Fresh fish

What do these food products have in common? They are all naturally occurring. The key, though, is to eat them in their natural state, or close to it. Don't substitute them with a quinoa health bar or a fish vitamin. This list does not include an energy drink made from blueberry extract. None of them, except some brands of tofu, come prepackaged with an expiration date or a nutrition label. And they don't need to be promoted by an infomercial

34

(meaning they're a lot less expensive than products that can turn a hefty profit.)

Here is the great diet secret revealed:

EAT REAL FOOD!

Preoperative Sleeve Knowledge Test II

Preoperative Sleeve Knowledge Test II (Quiz)

I should:

a. *Keep my weight loss efforts a secret.*

b. *Tell everybody I am having gastric sleeve surgery.*

c. *Understand that social support is very important to my long-term success.*

I should:

a. *Eat only liquids and mushy foods that go down easily.*

b. *Try to eat small amounts of nutritious foods.*

c. *Take one last bite after I feel full, just to be sure.*

When it comes to vitamins after gastric sleeve surgery,

a. *I should become a Flintstones Kid!*

b. *I don't have to take any because you just pee them out anyway.*

c. *I will take a multivitamin designed for bariatric patients for at least one year, and then get my nutrients from eating a wide variety of fresh fruits and vegetables.*

After surgery,

a. *I will need to take an antacid medicine, like Protonix because of the increased acid production.*

b. *I will need to have an upper endoscopy in two years to check out my sleeve anatomy.*

c. *I will need regular blood work.*

d. *All of the above*

Name six sources of protein.

Preoperative Sleeve Knowledge Test II (Answers)

I should:

a. *Keep my weight loss efforts a secret.*

False. Have you ever dieted in secret? How did that work out for you? Let me guess—not so great. That's probably because the people around you expected you to stick to your established patterns and offered you your favorite foods or urged you to indulge at your favorite restaurants. You had no one to talk with when the diet became difficult to maintain, nobody knew anyway, and so you probably quit.

> *The key to weight loss success is adherence.*

We encourage our patients to find their support people and enlist their help. Like The Beatles' famous song says, we could all use a little help from our friends. Maybe you didn't tell your friends or family because you were afraid that you would fail. If you think that you might fail before you even begin, you probably will. It is difficult to stick to long-term goals, and so you must not allow failure to be an easy option. Make it harder to quit than to keep going by letting those close to know what you are trying to accomplish. Then, when things become difficult, they can help keep you on track. And because admitting failure is never pleasant, even when you're alone, you will probably try harder.

b. *Tell everybody I am having gastric sleeve surgery.*

Not necessarily everybody. I wish every one of my patients would shout, "I had my gastric sleeve surgery with Dr. Vuong!" But having weight loss surgery is a private decision. If you are not ready to share your surgical experience with people you know, then you can try to say things like, "I'm just trying to make better choices for my health!" Hopefully, others will be respectful of your new lifestyle and encourage you to be even healthier.

I have found that it is almost impossible to keep word about your surgery from getting out. Even if your spouse remains quiet on the subject, you still need to ask for time off from work. Coworkers will just naturally be curious to know what you are doing so they will know how to help you. Your family and close friends will want to come visit you in the hospital; and people from church will wonder why you're not at service, etc...In the end, people are going to know. So I suggest to my patients that they take control over this aspect of their life and ask for the support of their closest friends and family. You will be surprised at who says what about your decision to have weight loss surgery, which gives you real insight into whom your real support people are.

c.   *Understand that social support is very important to my long-term success.*

Very true! Our society is built around food and eating. Everybody has an Aunt Patty who says, "I knew you were coming, so I baked you your favorite—pecan pie!" Aunt Patty is not trying to sabotage your weight loss efforts, but rather is trying to welcome you into her home. If you don't let Aunt Patty know about your new lifestyle beforehand, in this situation, you will either unhappily undermine your weight loss efforts or upset your relative. In order to achieve long-term, meaningful, weight loss happiness, you must have social support, which is why I recommend that my patients tell everyone about their surgery.

Every patient is so excited about their surgery date. The perioperative period (the time around the date of your surgery) is the easy part. I tell my patients,

> *"It's the living afterwards that's hard."*

You will have a lifetime of roadblocks and hurdles, temptations and struggles, supporters and naysayers. So set yourself up for success before surgery: identify your critical support personnel.

I should:

a. Eat only liquids and mushy foods that go down easily.

False. The gastric sleeve is not designed to stop liquids. In fact, if liquids can't go down, then you are in a lot of trouble! Eating only liquids is not a good long-term option, and consuming too many calories in the form of liquids is an easy trap. Consumption of liquid calories, like soda, is one of the major contributors to the current obesity epidemic. I consider ice cream, refried beans, and other soft and fatty foods along the same lines as liquids because the sleeve does not slow them down and they add far too many calories to your diet. Relatively speaking, they are too high in calories and too low in nutrition. Many people do not meet their weight loss goals because they are unwilling to give up high calorie drinks (including alcohol). You've got to decide which you want more—to be healthier and thinner or to have that soda. Decide this before you have your surgery. If you don't think that you can give up soda, the surgery will not help you.

Diet sodas are not an option either. Study after study has shown that people who consume the most diet sodas also tend to be the heaviest. Soda, diet or not, provides you with absolutely no nutrients. Read the ingredients—do you recognize many of them as food? In addition to doing nothing healthy for you, the chemicals in the diet soda accustom our palate to unnaturally sweet flavors, meaning that they encourage us to consume more sugar overall. I believe this is true with artificial sweeteners in your coffee, in your baking, anywhere. I don't care what color packet they come in—pink, blue, yellow, or any new color— artificial sweeteners are bad for you and encourage you to eat more sugary foods.

Some people think that shakes are good, and while it is true that high protein, low-calorie shakes have their role in the life of a weight loss surgery patient, shakes should not be relied upon for lasting weight-loss happiness. A smoothie made from fresh berries is great after a long day in the garden, but I want you to ...

> *Learn to eat and enjoy real food again.*

b. *Try to eat small amounts of nutritious foods.*

True. I tell all of my weight loss surgery patients that they should eat three, small, nutritious meals a day. Diabetics should also add a healthy snack. But what is "nutritious" or "healthy"? This is where the LOVE OF LEARNING comes in handy. A simpler way of thinking about this is to give your food the caveman test. For example, rotisserie chicken is nutritious, and a caveman would recognize a roasted bird. He would definitely not recognize chicken nuggets or the containers of sauce to dip them in. So choose the chicken that's been grilled or roasted, but leave behind the battered, processed, sauced-up varieties.

Most patients know that the first rule of weight loss surgery is "Protein first." But in my quest to teach my patients proper nutrition, I have created two additional RULES OF WEIGHT LOSS SURGERY, which we will discuss in the next quiz. I believe these two new rules have dramatically improved my patients' success.

c. *Take one last bite after I feel full, just to be sure.*

False. "One last bite" gets a lot of weight loss surgery patients into trouble. Learn to listen to your sleeve's cues to stop eating—and yes, these cues will change over time. Some patients get somatic clues, like a hiccup or a small burp, but not everyone does. And sometimes those clues will change as your body adapts to having a reduced stomach capacity.

If ever you are eating and think, **"Hmmm...maybe I should stop?"**, then guess what you should do? STOP EATING! It sounds simple, but I am always surprised by how many patients don't listen to this clue, especially if it is combined with a slight pressure in your chest. If you feel satisfied, you are done and there's no need to eat more. Food is plentiful here, and that last bite will do you more harm than good.

When it comes to vitamins after gastric sleeve surgery,

a. *I should become a Flintstones Kid!*

False. Early on, taking a simple multivitamin a day was the best advice we could give weight loss surgery patients, especially since they were chewable or came in liquid form. Now we know that this is not enough. So the vitamin industry has developed some bariatric-specific vitamins that are also great-tasting.

b. *I don't have to take any because you just pee them out anyway.*

False. This can be true if you take too much of one supplement, like consuming large amounts of vitamin C when you feel a cold coming on. But if you have had a gastric bypass, then you should definitely be taking multiple supplements every day.

c. *I will take a multivitamin designed for bariatric patients for at least one year, and then get my nutrients from eating a wide variety of fresh fruits and vegetables.*

True. We are just starting to understand what supplementation is needed after gastric sleeve surgery. Theoretically, since the sleeve does not involve any malabsorption, you shouldn't have to take vitamins and supplements forever. However, some studies are showing deficiencies in vitamin D as well as other trace elements. This does not mean that the gastric sleeve causes vitamin deficiencies; rather, I think it indicates how poor in nutrition our most common foods are.

I tell my patients to take bariatric-specific, nutritional supplements for one year after gastric sleeve surgery, but your surgeon's program might have different recommendations. For that first year, as my patients' diets change, I feel they need help nutritionally because it does take a while to learn to like new foods. I didn't like eggplant the first time I tried it, so I don't expect my patients to either. But they have to keep trying. Sometimes, it takes more than a year. It has taken me almost my entire life to learn to like some foods, such as tofu. Some things have come easier, like mushrooms and spinach. But patients have to try and they have to continue to try, just like I do.

After surgery,

a. *I will need to take an antacid medicine, like Protonix because of the increased acid production.*

True. Surgeons believe the gastric sleeve surgery is an acid-inducing procedure. At least initially, once a surgeon has removed about 75 % of your stomach, the remaining acid cells compensate for the missing 75 % by hyper-secreting acid. In other words, the remaining acid cells work harder to produce more acid because your body was used to producing a certain amount of acid prior to surgery. But you won't be able to eat as much food after your sleeve surgery to absorb all this acid. To help control this, most surgeons will put patients on a medication known as a proton pump inhibitor or PPI.

There is currently no standardization on how long patients need to be on this acid-blocker medication. Duke University keeps its patients on a PPI for one year. I suggest three months for my patients, because most of them don't need it after that. However, some continue to take it regularly for four to six months, and I have a few patients who still use it occasionally after one year.

b. *I will need to have an upper endoscopy in two years to check out my sleeve anatomy.*

True. I think some sort of imaging is necessary about two years after surgery. Think of it as routine maintenance for your sleeve, like a regular 25,000-mile service for your car. For my patients, I choose endoscopy. This allows me to accurately size and visualize my patient's sleeve. If I see anything unusual, I have the option of acting right then and there, like taking a biopsy. I can also show my patients actual pictures of their sleeves, which I find gives them some comfort knowing that everything is ok with their sleeve.

An x-ray study called a barium swallow is also helpful. It demonstrates the flow of liquid down your esophagus and through your sleeve into the small intestine. This could be very useful information, especially you are having problems.

c.   I will need regular blood work.

True. This is not specific to weight loss surgery patients. As part of a regular health check-up, everyone should get routine blood work done. Bariatric patients, however, need their blood checked for a few extra items. These are mostly vitamins and micronutrient levels that pertain more to gastric bypass patients. However, I think it is a good idea to check them in sleeve patients, too.

Every program is different. I recently attended a bariatric conference in Indianapolis, where I learned that one program runs an entire page of labs on its patients—some of which I hadn't even heard of before! I'm not saying it's right or wrong. While this is the most extreme example of blood work that I've encountered, every program will require some sort of regular blood work.

d.   All of the above

Name six sources of protein.

I will discuss the role of protein elsewhere, as well as how my conception of protein in the bariatric patient's diet has changed over the past several years. In the meantime, it is important to know natural sources of protein, especially non-animal based ones:

Vegetables—like broccoli

Beans—including lentils

Soy Products—tofu, edamame, and soy milk are great sources of protein with
    almost no fat

Whole Grains—couscous, bulgur and quinoa. Quinoa is being touted as the
    "perfect" protein source. I don't know if that will end up being true,
    but I do know that these grains are super easy to cook!

Nuts—like almonds and walnuts. Beware, though, because nuts are typically
    high in fat. I tell my patients that nuts from a tree (e.g., almonds,
    cashews, pecans, macadamias, piastachios, walnuts) are better than

nuts from the ground (e.g., peanut). I think that peanut butter is pretty much junk food, not much healthier than jam.

Fish—fresh, preferably wild-caught. I think freezing fish can sometimes alter its flavor and texture, and fish from a can is too processed. There are lots of varieties of fish, so find one you like. If you already like fish, that's great because it can be a healthy, lean source of protein that is versatile. It's ok if you don't currently like fish, but keep trying.

Chicken—even skinless, boneless chicken breast is too high in fat when compared to vegetables, grains, beans, and tofu. I don't think turkey is much better. I discuss this more fully in the Maintenance Section of the book.

Meat—beef is too high in fat. There is no such thing as a "lean cut" of meat. Maybe it's "leaner" compared to other cuts of meat, but it is still too high in fat. Pork is also a red meat, not "the other white meat." Game meat (such as venison) is better, but it can still be high in fat.

Dairy—no one should drink whole milk except for baby cows. I cover this in a Maintenance topic.

Prepackaged Protein Supplements—for convenience or as part of a perioperative program, protein shakes are ok on occasion. However, they should not form part of your daily or long-term diet. They are incomplete at best, and I think detrimental at worst. I recently saw an episode of "Shark Tank", one of the few television shows I like to watch, in which an entrepreneur was promoting a protein-enhanced water endorsed by a current football player. Really?

> *I tell my patients they can eat as much as they want from everything above the line, and sparingly from the food items below the line.*

If Americans did this one thing, I think we would cure or improve about 90% of our health problems.

Basic Nutrition Test

Basic Nutrition Test (Quiz)

What is the First Rule of Weight Loss Surgery (WLS) Eating?

What is the Second Rule of WLS Eating?

What is the Third Rule of WLS Eating?

How many calories per gram of Protein? Carbohydrate? Fat?

How many calories per gram of EtOH (alcohol)?

Why is this relationship important?

What two qualities define "Empty Calories"?

Give 3 examples of Empty Calorie foods.

How are these Empty Calorie Foods different from Super Foods?

Write one eating habit you still NEED to change.

Basic Nutrition Test (Answers)

What is the First Rule of Weight Loss Surgery (WLS) Eating?

FIRST RULE: Protein First!

These two little words mean a lot to bariatric patients. The rule teaches that at each meal, you should eat protein before you eat carbohydrates or fat. If your answer was "Chew, chew, chew" or "Don't drink during meals" or something like that, those are indeed good guidelines that you need to know. But make no doubt about it: the First Rule is "Protein First." Most patients' problems with weight loss and weight loss surgery can usually be traced back to the violation of this rule.

For the past few years and since writing my first book, I have backed away from stringent adherence to this rule. It is still important, but some surgeons and healthcare professionals are going overboard and pushing too much protein. Some programs are telling patients to eat 80 grams of protein a day. I believe that this is way too much! Your body probably can't process this much protein healthily. The "average" nonsurgical American woman only needs about 45 grams a day and man needs about 55 grams a day. The initial push for such high protein levels was due to the malabsorption that occurred with gastric bypass and duodenal switch patients. There is now an entire industry of protein shakes and protein "bullet shots," for example, that are trying to fill this demand. But it is not really needed because all of the protein we need is provided by our natural food sources, especially given our advances in surgery that lead to better absorption of nutrients.

While I still encourage patients to focus on eating protein first, I now take care to recommend the source of this protein. I instruct my patients to eat protein mostly from plant and fish sources and very little from animal sources, which are too high in fat. The cattle industry uses mostly corn for feed instead of allowing the animals to graze naturally. This has resulted in fattier meat, which many consumers prefer. This is often referred to as the "marbling" in a steak. Yet while the fat content has increased, the actual amount of protein in modern beef has decreased! The same is true for pork. So as a protein source, animal meat is not the best option.

> ### For BEST results, eat more non-animal sources of protein.

Now I think a vegan (pronounced VEE-gun) diet, when done properly, is probably the healthiest option, but it is hard to be a strict vegan in some areas of the country. A vegan is someone who chooses to avoid consuming or using animal products as a part of a healthy, environmentally-responsible, and cruelty-free lifestyle. In addition to not consuming meats, strict vegans also avoid dairy, eggs, and butter as well as fur, leather, wool, down, and cosmetics or chemical products tested on animals. There are many athletes (Arian Foster, running back for Houston Texans) and actors/actresses (Natalie Portman, *Black Swan*, *Star Wars* saga) who are vegans. And of course, lots of other individuals who lead similarly healthy and vibrant lives. Learn more about this fascinating and healthy option at www.vegan.org.

I am primarily a pescatarian (a vegetarian who eats seafood), but I also love a good steak every now and then; I just know I can't have it that often. Ultimately, I teach my patients to do the things that I do. I discuss this much more in the section titled "The Texture Scale."

What is the Second Rule of WLS Eating?

I soon realized the shortcomings of the First Rule, so I created two more rules. This next rule has made such a tremendous improvement in my patients' success and happiness that I have considered making it the #1 Rule:

SECOND RULE: Fill your pouch with the most nutritious food you can, most of the time.

With this rule, you must think of your sleeve as a long skinny pouch. This actually applies to everybody. Without surgery, your stomach is a big, floppy pouch, capable of stretching to hold 60 hot dogs, like the 4th of July eating contestants. Gastric band patients have a small pouch above their band, and gastric bypass patients have a small pouch that has been created by their surgeon. Your goal, if you want to be a healthy human being, is to fill that pouch with the most nutritious food you can, most of the time.

This rule works in coordination with the First Rule. Let's see how. We break down the Second Rule into three parts.

Part 1: Fill your pouch with protein first.

Why protein first? Protein sources are slower to digest and help patients have satiety for longer. "Slider foods," like chips, refried beans, and mashed potatoes, will not fill your pouch. They will slide right on through and defeat the purpose of weight loss surgery, which is to limit the amount you eat. Often weight loss surgery patients are surprised that they can eat an entire bag of chips after surgery. They cannot, however, eat the same amount of chicken as they did before. So choose protein first because it will fill your pouch longer and allow the surgery to work for you.

Also notice that I start the rule with the word "Fill". "Fill" is an action verb that places the responsibility on YOU to do what YOU need to do to be successful. It's not "I should" or "I will hope" or "I will try." It's not even "eat" or "drink," because after years of dieting, these words carry connotations that can be negative. Let's move outside our long-standing relationship with food and start thinking differently. You will FILL with nutritious food.

Part 2: With the most nutritious food you can→protein first

If you are eating your protein first, then I know that you are getting some form of nutrition. It might not be the best form, but some is better than none. The key word in this section is "nutritious." That means, now, you must think about the content of the foods you eat. What can a particular food do for you? In addition to making you feel full, protein can give you energy, repair sore muscles, and increase brain functioning. Can a milkshake do all those things? Can a dinner roll?

Learn what "NUTRITIOUS" means!

It's not enough to say, "But it's low-fat! Or fat-free! Or it's made by Lean Cuisine®, so it must be healthy!" Not true! YOU have to take the time and interest to learn what is meant by "nutritious." How do you do that? An easy clue comes from Rule #3, which we will discuss below.

Part 3: Most of the time→protein first

Why only MOST of the time? Why not be perfect ALL of the time? Because "life happens," and it will happen to you, too. There will always be birthdays and anniversaries and celebrations and reunions. On these occasions, it's ok to have fun—in any manner you wish, whether it includes food or not—but MOST of your days, you should make proper choices. If most of your meals include fresh fruits, vegetables, and lean protein, like fish, your body will keep running strong on the occasions when you don't give it good nutrition. It's not realistic to try and "be good" during holidays and celebrations. Has there ever been a time when you chose not to eat in front of people and left the party hungry, so later that evening you made a poor food choice and then felt guilty? Most patients have. I'm asking you to change that perspective. It's ok to have fun and splurge when the occasion calls for it, but in your day-to-day life, you should make mostly good choices. Decide what is worth celebrating. Your birthday and anniversary and major holidays are a few examples of occasions worth celebrating. Is your stepson's roommate's promotion? Is finishing work early on a Tuesday?

What is the Third Rule of WLS Eating?

THIRD RULE: You can eat all of the fresh fruits and vegetables you want, any time you want, as much as you want.

This is also known as **Kizzie's Rule**, named after my daughter. I developed this rule for her during meal times; then I realized how great it would be for my patients. Here is the story behind Kizzie's Rule:

I do the majority of the cooking in my household. Often, while I was chopping vegetables, Kizzie would come and ask me for some of what I was intending to cook, like a piece of carrot or slice of bell pepper. I always gladly gave her a few pieces, but one day, she came back and asked for more. My first reaction was to say, "But then we won't have enough for the entrée." I caught myself and realized how foolish it was that I would deny my daughter something so healthy, especially when parents all over America struggle with getting their kids to eat vegetables. So I gladly gave her the second helping. Now I plan ahead and buy extra vegetables just for her to eat before dinner, like an entire red bell pepper. Because I know she ate something healthy before dinner, I don't fuss if she doesn't want to eat her vegetables during dinner. This makes meal times much more relaxing, too!

Contrast this with the typical American family scenario, where the child says, "Mommy, I'm hungry. Can I have a banana?" The parent usually responds with, "No, because you'll ruin your dinner." But then what is dinner these days? Dinner is usually hamburgers, hot dogs, chicken nuggets, pizza, or macaroni and cheese. The child would have been better off nutritionally having a banana.

I refer to this as a **liberating rule**. For patients who have struggled and failed on multiple diets that were based on limitations and restrictions, Rule #3 is intended to liberate them, to open their world to a limitless variety of real food. If you are hungry at 10 in the morning, then Kizzie's Rule says you can have any piece of fruit, like strawberries. If your blood sugars are low at 4 in the afternoon, you can have carrots. If you are awake at midnight (why are you awake at midnight?), then Rule #3 says you can have ANY fresh fruit or vegetable you can think of. My family keeps a platter of fruit on a table for these occasions, as well as baby carrots. We have vines full of sweet tomatoes outside our back door. It can be fun trying out new produce, and your body will thrive on the vitamins and minerals! In addition, you can eat as much as you want without feeling guilty. Why is this? Because honestly, I've NEVER done a weight loss surgery on someone who ate too many fruits and vegetables. **No one has ever come into my office and said, "I'm overweight because I eat too much spinach."**

Think of Rule #3 as your ticket to a whole new world of foods. If your answer is, "What is so exciting about fruits and vegetables," or "I don't like vegetables," or "I grew up on a farm so I have already tried all of the vegetables there are," I would say that there are still vast varieties of fruits and vegetables your taste buds are waiting for you to discover. For example, have you ever tasted the juicy sweetness of a rambutan? What's the difference between dragon fruit, logan fruit, or jujubee fruit? Have you ever felt the sting of a bittermelon? Can you taste the subtle difference between dinosaur kale, mezuna, and wild rocket? Other than button, what varieties of mushrooms have you eaten? Have you tried porcini, oyster, shitake? The corollary to Kizzie's Rule is if you have never tried it, you can't say you don't like it. So go try something new today!

> *There are over 7500 varieties of apples in the world, but only one way to deep-fry.*

How many calories per gram of Protein? 4 Carbohydrate? 4 Fat? 9

"What does this question even mean, Dr. Vuong?" Well, imagine that the plastic cap for a bottle of water is one gram of protein. You eat the cap. How many calories of protein did you just eat? Answer is 4 calories. Now imagine it is one gram of carbohydrate and then one gram of fat. In each instance if you eat that one gram bottle cap, you would consume 4 and 9 calories respectively.

How many calories per gram of EtOH (alcohol)? 7

This is pure alcohol, not the TYPE of alcohol like wine vs. beer or tequila vs. vodka. It's not the alcoholic drink, like a White Russian. It is the actual alcohol compound that causes intoxication.

Why is this relationship important?

See Preoperative Knowledge Test I, Question #3 for more details, but basically, it means that for the same weight of food, you consume over twice the calories if you pick something fatty (like sausage) versus something with very little or no fat (like fish). Look at the next nutrition label you come across when comparing two food items—the item with more fat content will have more calories for the same serving size.

Another way to look at this relationship is that you can eat more than twice the amount of protein or carbohydrates as fat for the same amount of calories. One sausage has about the same amount of calories as twice the same weight of fish. Most diets try to encourage us to eat less. I often tell my patients that I am the only doctor they will ever meet who will tell them they can eat MORE, not LESS, but that WHAT they eat must change. In adopting weight loss surgery patients who had surgery elsewhere, I find that if a patient thought before surgery that she could eat the same thing after surgery, but just less of it, and has not changed her food choices, then she is probably struggling with her weight loss. With that way of thinking, I can almost guarantee that they have stopped losing weight and are still overweight or have started regaining their weight.

This caloric relationship also means that those alcoholic drinks can add a lot of calories (and no nutrients) to your intake without helping you feel full, especially mixed drinks where the calories come more from the mixer or ingredients than from the alcohol itself, because the drink consists mostly of the mixer. For example, a White Russian has vodka, a sweet coffee liqueur like Kahlua, and cream. So it's easy to see that the majority of calories will be from the cream and the coffee liqueur. "But Dr. Vuong, White Russians are sooo good!" I agree they are tasty, but I tell my patients that if they choose to drink a White Russian, just accept the fact that you will probably not lose weight for the next two days. And that's ok. The problem is when people think that somehow a rum and Diet Coke® is a good weight loss alternative, when it's not.

What two qualities define "Empty Calories"?

They are the scurge of every WLS patient, regardless of the type of procedure you've had. Empty calories are foods that are HIGH in calories, but LOW in nutrition. They are the usual culprits when I hear or read about a "weight loss plateau."

> **HIGH IN CALORIES + LOW IN NUTRITION = WEIGHT LOSS DISASTER**

Remember to think about what foods can do for you, and those empty calories won't seem so appealing. They are lazy calories that just lie around and don't do any work for our bodies.

Give 3 examples of Empty Calorie foods.

Ice cream, soft drinks, candy bars, chips, and nearly every highly processed food that resides in a snack machine. I would even say most fast foods are nothing but empty calories. Their low nutritional value does not justify their high caloric counts. Sadly, these are often the most convenient foods. A small "snack" from the machines at work can take just seconds and a few coins to purchase, but may contain a few hundred calories that sap you of your energy and rob you of your goals.

These "convenient food items" are so low in nutrition that I don't even consider them food. Food is meant to nourish our bodies. If a food item is nourishing—i.e. full of nutrients—then mold and bacteria will quickly decompose it. If mold will eat it, then the food will spoil.

> ### *Real food should spoil.*

A lot of the processed products Americans eat will not spoil! Did you ever wonder why a Cheeto you find between your couch cushions two months later still looks the same? The bag of popcorn still looks appetizing a year later? These are not foods; they are processed chemicals. Is that what you want fueling your body or the bodies of your children?

How are these Empty Calorie Foods different from Super Foods?

Empty calorie foods are readily available, quickly consumed, and come in convenient packaging. Super foods take more effort to find, challenge your taste buds, and have their own natural packaging. The packaging of empty calorie foods pollutes our environment and adds to our landfills. The packaging of super foods is usually edible or biodegradable. Empty calorie foods are often man-made. Super foods are usually nature-made—they come out of the ground, grow on a bush, or hang from a tree.

Only two things will survive a nuclear holocaust—empty calorie foods and roaches. Super foods will spoil. Empty calorie foods are full of chemical preservatives; super foods have natural antioxidants and nutrition that help you preserve your health. Food scientists create combinations that make empty calorie foods addictive, that take you on sugar highs and then crash you down. Super foods are created by Mother Nature and are naturally addictive because of the super way they make you feel when you eat them. Super foods are not just addictive; they are necessary. Your body will work and feel better if you start replacing empty calorie "food" with super food.

Empty calorie foods destroy your dreams. Super foods will give you the energy to pursue your dreams.

> ### *Empty calories are the enemy.*

Vanquish your enemy from your lands.

Write one eating habit you still NEED to change.

The great motivational speaker Jim Rohn is famous for saying, "In order for things to change, YOU MUST change. If you don't change, then nothing will change. IF you will change, EVERYTHING will change for you."

My life changed the day I heard these words, so I pass on this message to you now. I cannot impress upon you enough how deeply this statement affected my thought processes. Every day, I strive to improve and get better. Every day, I let the failures of yesterday go and look forward to the challenges of today. I hope you will do the same. It is a powerful shift in mindset. It gives you back control of your life. I have many bad habits, but I try to improve one habit at a time. I am not always successful, but I keep trying. I hope you will keep trying too.

The Texture Scale™

The Texture Scale™ (Quiz)

Fill in the Texture Scale below.

The left side, designated by #1, is the thinnest texture, such as that of water. The right side of the scale (#6) is the thickest texture, which is that of steak. Figure out what food items make up the remaining scale; e.g., for #2, what is slightly thicker in texture than water? Here are some items you might consider for the scale: pork, fish, bread, chicken, vegetables, shakes, shrimp.

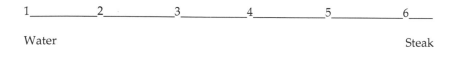

1_____2_____3_____4_____5_____6____

Water   Steak

How is the Texture Scale useful?

What does the scale *not* tell us about our food choices?

How does the Texture Scale relate to the Three Rules?

First Rule: Protein First

Second Rule: Fill your pouch with the most nutritious food you can most of the time.

Third Rule: You can eat all of the fresh fruits and vegetables you want anytime you want.

Where does "bread" go on the Texture Scale; i.e., what texture number would you assign to bread?

What is "Mushy Food Syndrome"?

Where on the Texture Scale should you be eating most of the time if you want to lose the most weight and have the most energy?

The Texture Scale™ (Answers)

Fill in the Texture Scale below.

The left side, designated by #1, is the thinnest texture, such as that of water. The right side of the scale (#6) is the thickest texture, which is that of steak. Figure out what food items make up the remaining scale; e.g., for #2, what is slightly thicker in texture than water? Here are some items you might consider for the scale: pork, fish, bread, chicken, vegetables, shakes, shrimp.

1_____2_____3_____4_____5_____6_____

Water   Steak

I created the Texture Scale to help my gastric band patients through their post-operative course. I also use it to help them during their adjustment process. (After an adjustment, I encourage my patients to be on liquids for a day and slowly progress through thicker textures to test the appropriateness of the adjustment.) Once I began performing gastric sleeves, I quickly realized that the Texture Scale is also a very helpful tool for sleeve patients.

In my groups, I have my patients go through the process of filling in the scale. It's not always intuitive, especially for the newer patients, but thinking carefully about food textures is helpful. Let's go through this process together now.

What do you think goes into space #2?

1_____2_____3_____4_____5_____6_____

Water **Mushy Foods**   Steak

Most patients will guess something like soup, pudding, or shakes, and these are all correct. I like to place such items into a category I call "Mushy Foods." Here are a few more Mushy Foods: mashed potatoes, creamed soups, yogurt, refried beans, and vegetables that have been super-boiled, to name a few.

In general, these foods are low in nutrition but high in calories. Immediately after surgery, my patients are on liquid Optifast for one week. Over the course of the second week after surgery, they slowly add mushy foods. I know that some surgery programs keep their patients on soft foods for a few weeks or even months, but I do not want my patients to stay on mushy foods for very long. I encourage my patients to add foods slowly and conscientiously, and when in doubt, to lean more on Optifast than on mushy foods. Optifast and other shakes tend to have more balanced nutrition than mushy foods do. I will talk more about the harms of staying on mushy foods too long below.

What do you think goes into space #3?

1_____2_____3_____4_____5_____6_____

Water   Mushy Foods   **Fish**   Steak

Space #3 is reserved for the mighty Fish and her powerful friends.

Among Fish's friends are fresh Fruit and Vegetables.

When prepared well, Fish is often described as "flaky." That slightly translucent texture should resonate clearly in your mind's eye. It should be reminiscent of Fish's close cousin—the firm, sweet flesh of Fruit. If you imagine the soft give of a ripe peach, Bartlett pear, or watermelon, you should agree that the textures of Fish and Fruit are very similar. Of course, a crisp apple, especially with the skin on, does not provide the same experience. Crisp apples and firm pears would rank more of a 3.5. Herein lies one of the truths of the Texture Scale: it is a *relative* scale. An overcooked fish might rank above a three, and soups laden with croutons would be much higher than a two. There are no hard-and-fast rules; it's the process of thinking about the relative textures of foods along the scale that will help you choose the foods that will work well with your surgery.

Most fresh vegetables also belong in category 3. Think bell pepper, squash, steamed broccoli florets, tomatoes, or spinach leaves. Do not think of the fibrous celery stalk. Cooked carrots, yes, but raw carrots...probably not. Focus on the nuances of the texture of the food, not the food itself.

What is #4?

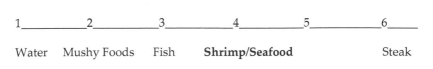

Water   Mushy Foods   Fish   **Shrimp/Seafood**   Steak

#4 is Shrimp and Other Seafood.

This includes delectable items, such as scallops, lobster, crab, and calamari. Why is shrimp thicker than fish? When fish is cooked well it is described as "nice and flaky," but overcooked shrimp is "rubbery" or "chewy". And most restaurants overcook shrimp. People are often surprised to learn that shrimp should be boiled for only about 6 minutes. Like fish, shrimp should also be cooked to a slight translucency at its center. Even then its texture is slightly thicker than fish's. This applies to other seafood also, such as scallops, lobster, and crab. Calamari and squid possess a slightly firmer texture, so they would rate around a 4.5. I've often wondered about raw oysters and the gastric sleeve. I would think that smaller oysters would be ok, but the Texas Gulf Coast oysters are so large, I'd be afraid that they may not be compatible with the sleeve.

As always, beware of the omnipresent "Friday Special": the Fried Seafood Platter. Not only has fresh seafood been tortured into something unhealthy, the batter masks the textural differences of the food.

Now, what is #5?

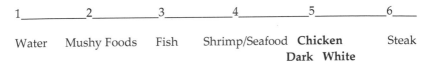

Water   Mushy Foods   Fish   Shrimp/Seafood **Chicken**   Steak
                                          Dark   White

Space #5 is occupied by every dieter's favorite—chicken!

Under chicken, there are two possible choices: dark or white meat. Which one do you suppose is thinner? Why? Dark meat is thinner, because it is slightly higher in fat and therefore juicier. White meat is thicker because it is drier and lower in fat. Which one of the two do you reckon I recommend for my weight loss surgery patients?

I tell my patients that if they don't already, then they should start choosing DARK meat! This might come as a surprise to several of the veteran dieters out there who cut their teeth (literally and figuratively) on skinless, boneless chicken breast. Here is my rationale:

- Most of the fat in chicken is actually in the skin, not the meat.
- Dark meat makes up for its slightly higher fat content by having more iron, which every young woman and many of the rest of us need.
- After weight loss surgery, you want to choose healthy foods that will not complicate your life. I can almost guarantee that at some point the weight loss surgery patient will get a piece of white meat chicken stuck, especially if it has been reheated.

So choose dark meat. If you don't like chicken legs or thighs, then I recommend that you learn to like it. It's like kale, broccoli, or tofu. You should learn to like it if you plan to be a meat-eater.

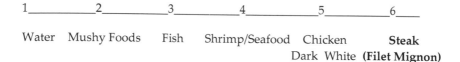

1	2	3	4	5	6
Water	Mushy Foods	Fish	Shrimp/Seafood	Chicken	**Steak**
				Dark White	**(Filet Mignon)**

As previously stated, #6 is Steak. But not all steaks are created equal!

If you are going to eat steak, you should choose the best cut: filet mignon. Why? Not because it is leaner but because you are worth it.

Choose Filet Mignon, because you are worth it!

If you don't like filet mignon, then choose the best cut of what you like, be it porterhouse, T-bone, or New York strip. Why pick the best? Because you will not be eating it very often and should enjoy it when you do. A typical filet will weigh eight ounces, and you will probably only be able to eat one or two ounces. The remaining six can go to your spouse, child, or friend. They're worth it, too!

Let's say you are at a very nice restaurant and the eight-ounce filet dinner you've ordered is $32. That is only $4 an ounce. If you eat two ounces plus a few bites of sides, then your meal was only $8. Are you not worth $8? Is your spouse or child not worth $24? This may seem silly, since you're spending

$32, no matter how much you eat, but why not split the plate with your dining companion?

Where do you think pork goes on the scale?

The answer is, "It depends." Pork is a red meat (no matter what the marketers say to the contrary), so in theory, it belongs with #6 Steak. But pork is very versatile. Did you slowly braise it for three hours until the pork fell off the bone? This might be a 5.5. Did your mother-in-law accidentally leave the pork cutlets in the oven too long, and now they are hard like hockey pucks? This would make them a 6.5 or 7 — or possibly even inedible.

> *Food texture changes depending on food preparation.*

This is true for the entire Texture Scale. The food items listed are not stagnant, but rather shift depending on the way they are prepared. The perfectly grilled fish will be a 3, but if you reheat that same fish the next day for lunch, it might be a 4 or 4.5. That tasty shrimp that went down easily last night might not do so well if you reheat it in the microwave. Most foods move up the texture scale when they are reheated, especially microwaved, because microwaves tend to sap the juices out of foods.

The only possible exceptions are soups (or stews) and meats that were braised and reheated it in their own broth. The extra liquid might keep the meats juicy. You just have to be cognizant of the texture as you are eating.

> *When you are chewing a piece of meat, and you get the sense that the meat is too tough, then just spit it out.*

This one tip could save you a long night in the emergency room and a trip to the endoscopy suite to remove the stuck mushy ball of meat.

How is the Texture Scale useful?

Even though I developed this scale initially for my gastric band patients, I now use it to teach my sleeve patients how to properly transition to thicker foods during their immediate postoperative period. During the weeks following sleeve surgery, the staple line is healing and needs protection from internal pressure. The swelling of the sleeve immediately after surgery can be so extreme that patients can often actually feel the slight textural difference between water and Optifast shakes. That slight increase in texture causes patients to feel pressure in their chests. So, think often of the Texture Scale when you start to add foods to your diet during the postoperative period and even well after surgery. You can also use the Texture Scale to help you plan your meals in your everyday life. If you know you're not ready for steak, then you probably are not ready for pork. If you know that you can have fish, then you can probably have that peach for a snack.

Broadly speaking, the Texture Scale indicates the quality of our food choices, too. The foods on the left side of the scale tend to be lower in nutritional value (think banana pudding, refried beans). The items on the right side of the scale are denser in texture but also higher in fat and, hence, calories. If you are eating a lot of Hamburger Helper and pork sausage, both of which fall on the right side of the scale, then you can surmise that your food choices have probably not been very lean; hence, your weight loss has probably not been optimal.

What does the scale *not* tell us about our food choices?

The Texture Scale does not grant carte blanche permission when it comes to selecting food. In other words, just because meat is on the scale, you shouldn't permit yourself to eat fast food hamburgers all of the time. The scale does not tell us about the nutritional quality of the food choices you make. You can't say, for example:

- "Well, since I got that filet mignon down, it's ok for me to have Taco Bell now."
- "Since I can only have mushies, I will blenderize a Snicker's bar."
- "Cheese is about the texture of fruit, so I will have string cheese everyday for a snack."
- "I'm on chicken, so chicken nuggets must be good for me."

These would not be good choices. The Texture Scale is to help you be deliberate about the food items you put into your body. Unlike "diets" that restrict your food choices, I offer you the opportunity to **expand your food horizons**, to explore and try different foods from different cultures, or as a famous commercial goes, to "think outside the box."

How does the Texture Scale relate to the Three Rules?

First Rule: Protein First

You should try to find the leanest sources of protein available, which will typically be fish and beans.

Question: Which item has the most protein: one ounce of fish, one ounce of chicken, one ounce of steak, or one ounce of cheese?

Answer: They all have about the same!

So what is the difference? **The fat content.** Fish has the least amount of fat, chicken is next, then meat, and finally cheese. We know that fat has more calories, so this means that meat and cheese are substantially higher in calories than fish. So for the same amount of protein and fewer calories, choose fish more often than meat. Or stated another way, for the same number of calories, you can eat a LARGER portion of fish and get MORE protein!

Second Rule: Fill your pouch with the most nutritious food you can most of the time.

There is no item labeled "junk" or "chips" on the scale. But again, just because the food item is listed, does not mean it is ok to eat. MOST of the time, you should be filling your pouch with nutritious foods. This means mostly fresh fruit, vegetables, and fish.

Third Rule: You can eat all of the fresh fruits and vegetables you want anytime you want.

This rule gives you the freedom that is lacking in most diets. The scale includes a nearly endless list of possible food choices.

"But Dr. Vuong, I'm tired of eating broccoli, carrot sticks, and apples!"

To which I reply, "Have you tried broccolini? How about mizuna or kale? What about Israeli cantaloupe, persimmons, or lychees? Did you know that Ambrosia, Pinata, and Cameo are only three of over 7500 varieties of apples? How many different varieties of bananas or tomatoes have you tried?" See, the choices are endless, and you can eat as many of these fruits and vegetables as you want.

In contrast, most junk foods are just the same corn-based, highly-processed goop, molded into different shapes, infused with different chemicals to add the missing "flavor," and stuffed into different packages.

Where does "bread" go on the Texture Scale; i.e., what texture number would you assign to bread?

Most patients guess bread is about a 3 or 4 on the Texture Scale. Some think it is a 6 or 7 because it can expand and get stuck and must therefore be thicker than steak.

My answer is that it is a trick question: **Bread is not on the scale.** Bread and all of the related processed white flour products have no place on the scale. You should consider it junk for the most part. Yes, it can get stuck, but it can also go down easily. It can be soft like sandwich bread or crusty like toast. But trust me, in America in the 21st century, bread is not your weight loss friend!

What is "Mushy Food Syndrome"?

Mushy foods are also called "slider foods," because they tend to "go down easily." A lot of weight loss surgery patients, especially banded patients, think this is a good thing, but it is not. Mushy foods are typically high in calories, but low in nutrition. I STRONGLY advise that you do not get hooked on eating mushy foods, like mashed potatoes and pudding. Here's why:

- What is your WEIGHT going to do if you eat mostly foods that are high in calories and low in nutrition?
  - o Answer: Plateau or increase
- What is your ENERGY LEVEL going to be like if you eat mostly foods that are high in calories and low in nutrition?
  - o Answer: Remain low so you feel sluggish

- What is your ATTITUDE going to be like if you eat mostly foods that are high in calories and low in nutrition?
  - Answer: Not very pleasant! Why? Because, "Dr. Vuong, I'm barely eating, I have no energy, and gosh darn it, I'm not even losing any weight!"

This cycle of poor choices/poor results is what I call the "Mushy Food Syndrome." You must avoid it at all costs if you want to be successful with weight loss.

Where on the Texture Scale should you be eating most of the time if you want to lose the most weight and have the most energy?

Hopefully, everything I've said so far makes sense to you and you can figure out the answer. For my patients (and for myself), I teach them to try and stay around the 3 to 4 range MOST of the time, with occasional forays into 5 to 6 (see the 21x Guide). The exception, of course, is water. Drink as much of it as you like!

Meat should remain a small side dish.

In Appendix B: The Texture Scale, I put it all together for you. Turn there now to see the Texture Scale in its final version.

How Do You Know When You Are Full?

How Do You Know When You Are Full? (Quiz)

How many times a day SHOULD you eat after weight loss surgery and why?

If you have not had your surgery, what do you imagine FULL will feel like?

If you have had surgery, how do you know when you are full?

What will happen to you if you ignore your "full" signal?

If something gets "stuck", what should you do?

What should you NOT do when food is stuck?

What is the Second Rule of WLS Eating?

How Do You Know When You Are Full? (Answers)

How many times a day SHOULD you eat after weight loss surgery and why?

I recommend that my patients eat at least **three small meals** a day, with each meal containing some protein (remember the First Rule?). I also tell my diabetics that they should add a fourth small snack in the afternoon to keep their blood sugars level, and by "snack" I do not mean candy, cookies, or other such sweet snacks (remember the Second Rule?). A small apple, a handful of blueberries, or a banana would do great (remember the Third Rule?)! High-sugar foods do not keep blood sugars even, but rather send them on a roller-coaster ride (remember that your food should work FOR you?).

Here is a lesson from a Lap-Band® patient. She is a dedicated employee and often gets to work early. Like most patients, she never ate anything for breakfast. She then would work through lunch and by the time she got home in the late evenings, she would be ravenous! Of course, then she would overeat on calorie-dense foods, like pasta or fast food. After she got the Lap-Band, she told us that the band was not keeping her satisfied, she was hungry all day, etc. After we went through her daily food intake, we discovered that she still patterned her meals the same way, but now because of the band, she could no longer eat a large amount in the evenings and she still did not eat at all during the day—thus her constant hunger! We reiterated the importance of eating small meals (Second Rule—Fill your pouch). I instructed her to have a convenient protein shake and small banana on her drive to work, a small meal for lunch like lentils and a salad, then dinner when she got home. She voiced understanding of the importance of proper eating throughout the day, but continued to make excuses for her inability to "find time" due to her "hectic work schedule." (I'm pretty busy, but I can still find time every day to eat a banana or grab a salad from the cafeteria, even if I can't go to a restaurant for a leisurely meal with friends.) To this day, I don't think she has made those changes and therefore has not been as successful as she had hoped.

I like this story because it demonstrates several points:

First, if you don't change your behaviors, you'll get the same results you always have.

Secondly, you need to KNOW the Three Rules.

Lastly, you've got to FOLLOW the Three Rules.

There are only three! I've been able to condense everything you need to know down to three rules, but ultimately YOU'VE got to follow them!

If you have not had your surgery, what do you imagine FULL will feel like?

Patients who expect their weight loss surgery, regardless of the type of surgery, to perform miracles rarely change their eating behaviors. Needless to say, these patients often are disappointed with their weight loss, find themselves stuck on a "weight loss plateau" (a concept that we do not believe in at my clinic), or regain a lot of their weight. While it is true that if you do not consume enough calories, your body's metabolism will slow down, this rationale for unsuccessful weight loss has been grossly exaggerated. The truth is that the vast majority of patients who are not losing weight are consuming too many empty calories. It is very hard to resist calorie-dense foods if you go too long between meals or if you have never changed the choices you make.

For example, I have a patient who eats anything chocolate when she is stressed, and I mean anything. Well, in September 2008, Hurricane Ike blew right over my surgical practice and house. The storm's track on the radar went right through my living room. She was a landlord, and it also damaged many of her rental properties. Needless to say, this really stressed her out, and she put on a lot of weight. But to her credit, she came back to our support groups and talked about her weight regain and stress. After a couple of weeks, she revealed how she used chocolate to alleviate her stress (she ate anything chocolate every night), but she could not see the connection between this empty calorie consumption and her weight regain. It's only a FEW pieces of chocolate," she'd say. I suggested that instead of consuming lots of whatever chocolate she could find, she should become a chocolate connoisseur and eat only the finest chocolates. I told her there were entire online communities and books about fine chocolate. She took my advice, and the following week had limited her chocolate consumption to only one evening and one portion of a very expensive chocolate bar. She lost two pounds that week! I was delighted that she was able to find a way to adapt this passion/addiction/stress-management technique into a much healthier approach. I was even happier when she gave all of the credit of this success to talking about it in support group.

Most things I hear from frustrated patients ("I'm too busy," "I can't find time to cook or exercise," "I can't get time off from work," etc.) boil down to one thing: they are all EXCUSES. As mean as that sounds, it's the truth. You are not the busiest person in the world (rather, you choose not to be as efficient in your work as you could be or choose to be busy with inessential activities). You are not the most stressed out person in the world (are you more stressed out then, say, our thin and fit President?) You are not the world's worst cook (there are marinated chicken breasts at the grocery store that you can just pop in the oven) or cannot exercise because of arthritis pain (there are many forms of exercise that do not require stress on joints.) These are just excuses that are used to justify not having to make a change. There are tips and techniques to accommodate ALL of these reasons. YOU just have to decide that YOU want to be healthier and happier MORE than you want that cookie or hour of television. And you do that by first changing the excuses you tell yourself in your head.

Let's go through some useful tips meal by meal. Remember that your goal is to fill your pouch with the most nutritious food you can most of the time.

BREAKFAST: Many Lap-Band patients complain of difficulty swallowing in the mornings. This is thought to be due to the thick mucus that builds up during the night. Try to alleviate this by drinking a cup of hot tea to break up the mucus. This is not as common in sleeve or gastric bypass patients. Nonetheless, some patients insist that they just "can't eat breakfast." I always ask them exactly what they mean by breakfast. The response usually is, "I can't eat pancakes with syrup and bacon and potatoes, etc." And I say, "Of course not!" The concept of a "meal" is different after weight loss surgery. You will not be able to eat a Denny's Grand Slam Breakfast anymore. But then why would you want to? That is a meal high in calories and fat and low in nutrition. It is too bad that meals like it have come to represent the American breakfast when there are many better options.

I recommend that my patients have a small, sensible breakfast, which for me, usually means a big glass of water and a piece of fruit. If they can't do that, then I recommend that they drink a high protein shake (like Optifast), understanding that this will pass right through their pouch into the remainder of their digestive tract, and then (and this is the key) they must fill their pouch with something nutritious like some Greek yogurt, 1/3 of a banana, or a nutrition bar. The protein shake will ensure that they get their protein, and the real food will help them control their hunger. And all of these options take a lot less time to prepare and eat than that stack of pancakes!

LUNCH: Your employer is usually required by law to give you a lunch break—30 minutes in most states. This is your right! Take it, and use it for lunch rather than errands, because it will mean everything to your success. You MUST eat lunch. I can't stress this enough. I really believe that it is by far the most important meal of the day. If you have a job in which you don't get a lunch break, make sure to keep some healthy and easy-to-eat foods handy, like a peach, carrot sticks, or a preboxed salad, and eat them a few hours after your breakfast. Surely you can find a few minutes to take a few bites.

> *Lunch is the most important meal, not breakfast!*

Prepare your lunch the night before if you can and bring it with you to work, so that you will be sure to have a nutritious meal handy. If you say that you don't have time to make your lunch, then I ask you, "Aren't you worth the extra 10 minutes it would take?" Or you can do what my partner does—make a quick lunch while the coffee brews in the morning. Many grocery stores have prepackaged fancy salads with all the trimmings and styles, like a Santa Fe salad or an Asian salad, and usually for under $5! If you choose to go with coworkers out to lunch, suggest a healthier restaurant choice. If they won't change their plans, don't go. Or, if you do go, then make a healthier choice by focusing on a low-fat, lean-protein selection that has mostly fresh vegetables, like a spinach salad topped with grilled shrimp, salmon, or chicken. Look for the "light and fit" portion of the menu.

DINNER: Learn to cook real food! This means buying fresh ingredients, including fresh vegetables, fruits, and meats. Anything you make is better than anything you can purchase from a fast food restaurant if you are using fresh ingredients. If all you have to do is pry open a can or tear open a cardboard box and heat it in the microwave, you are probably not making the best choice. That's not real cooking. Refried beans from a can are usually no better than refried beans in a Tex-Mex restaurant, which are often from a can anyway. If it has shelf life, it's not fresh (think back to the caveman). I don't care if it says Lean Cuisine® or Healthy Choice® on the box—that's all advertising, and don't fall for it! Learn five simple recipes with fresh ingredients and start from there. Watch cooking shows, read magazines, or pick up a cookbook from a bookstore. I love to cook now, but I didn't start off that way. I've ruined and have had to throw away plenty of groceries to get to this point. But it's worth the effort, and your first attempts don't have to be fancy or complicated. Make no mistake about it: **cooking fresh is best**.

I bet if you stopped and added up the cost of all of the cans and boxes of "food" you have in your pantry, you'd be shocked at how much you've spent. Why else do people have to have a walk-in pantry or an extra freezer for meat storage? In the 21st century in America, we have ready access to food. We really don't need all these empty calories lying around "just in case." I call that the "Just in Case" Syndrome. Just in case company comes over. Just in case I am late getting home from work. Just in case I have to babysit the grandchildren. Just in case a nuclear war breaks out...

> *Don't fall for the "Just in Case" Syndrome.*

With storage, every food item loses the quality of its natural flavor. To make up for this, food companies add flavorings and preservatives, which is a fancy way of saying acceptable levels of unnatural chemicals. So when you cook, choose just enough of the freshest and best quality produce that is the main ingredient or ingredients for your meal. The result will taste a lot better and be a lot healthier.

If you have had surgery, how do you know when you are full?

Instead of feeling full in their belly, most patients report experiencing a "pressure feeling" right in the middle of their chest. They are confused by the location of this feeling. I tell them that that is where their band is sitting, where the gastric sleeve starts, or where their gastric bypass pouch begins. Many are surprised to learn this. So I explain it like this: Most surgeons will use a liver retractor to access the gastroesophageal junction (GEJ). This is the area of the stomach where all surgeons eventually have to visualize, regardless of the procedure. If you look at your surgical scars, you should have a small scar in the upper middle, where both sides of your rib cage come together at your sternum or "breastbone." That little area is called your xiphoid. Put your finger on this scar and move up one inch. Then imagine a line going from your finger to your back. This imaginary line will hit your band, the start of your sleeve, or your gastric pouch. Yes, your surgery is that high up! And that is why you get the pressure feeling in your chest and not around your belt line like before.

After weight loss surgery, you won't feel "Thanksgiving full" anymore. Before having surgery, most patients expect to feel like they just had second helpings of a big turkey dinner after every meal, but that is just not the case. You won't need to unbuckle your belt, sit in the recliner, and watch the Cowboys' game. But why would you want that feeling after every meal? I compare it to when you, a busy and stressed-out person, imagine how wonderful it would be to be able to stay in bed all day. But having taken care of people who are bed-bound, I will tell you that bed confinement gets really old really fast. I imagine experiencing that heavy fullness after every single meal would get old even faster! Instead, your meals should leave you feeling satisfied and energized.

Some patients report feeling pain in their back or between their shoulder blades after eating too much after surgery. The location of this discomfort is again close to where the surgery took place. I have one patient who gets a small burp, which is her signal to stop eating. I have several band patients who will hiccup—this is probably due to irritation of the diaphragm muscles when their pouch is full. My sleeve patients get more of the pressure or tightness sensation. These sorts of signals can help recent surgery patients learn to recognize fullness.

While these signals are convenient, not everyone gets them. Don't be disappointed if you don't have a signal or haven't recognized it yet. It is so much more important to learn the feeling of SATIETY. It is OK to be satisfied. (It's what Mick Jagger has been looking for all these years.) Stop eating when you are satisfied, not stuffed. This is often the most difficult part for many patients, many of whom do not know what it means to be satisfied. If you eat regular meals, you have no reason to become stuffed, because you'll eat again in a few hours. Overeating is often a way to compensate for going far too long between meals. Instead of eating to try to ward off future hunger, try instead to only worry about feeling satisfied now. There will be plenty of food later for when you feel hungry again.

Since the writing of my last book, here is one stance I've become more dogmatic about:

It's not natural to be full.

It's natural to be hungry.

But Americans ALWAYS want to feel full and NEVER want to be hungry. If you think about it, this is basically the promise of every diet out there. "If you follow our diet (take our pill, sprinkle our dust, drink our shake), you will feel fuller faster and not get hungry between meals," or something to that effect. I'm here to tell you, these diets will not work long-term (and perhaps you have discovered this after trying several of them). The reason is because it is natural for our bodies to get hungry (it's our way of knowing it's time for nourishment) and it is unnatural for us to feel full all of the time (food was just too scarce as we were evolving). We had to hunt and gather our foods. We ate fresh ingredients that were provided by Mother Earth. And notice I used the phrase "time for nourishment" as opposed to "time to eat." It is more important for your body's overall functioning for it to be nourished than for it to be full. I discuss this important idea in more detail later in the section entitled "The Truth About Hunger".

What will happen to you if you ignore your "full" signal?

It's like what Clubber Lang, a.k.a Mr. T, told the reporter in Rocky III: "Pain." You will feel SEVERE PAIN IN YOUR CHEST, like you are having a heart attack. And there is not much that you can do about it. Below are the typical experiences after food items have gotten stuck for each different procedure:

- Gastric Band—I find stuck food episodes are more common with the band than other procedures because the gastric band for whatever reason can be "finicky." Its temperament may be due to the way the surgeon placed the band, the size of the band, the follow-up care provided, and patient behaviors. But these episodes should be few and far between, as long as you stay well adjusted. However, if you never go back for an adjustment (or unadjustment), the fluid in the band will very slowly seep out over the years, and it will be as if you've never even had the surgery.

- Gastric Sleeve—If you overeat once with the sleeve, I bet you will not do it again. I find the sleeve is very compatible with regular, everyday socializing. On only a few occasions has one of my sleeve patients gotten an item stuck, usually around the immediate postoperative period, as the patient was transitioning through different textured foods. The impacted food item will usually pass on its own, but occasionally it will come back up.

- Gastric Bypass—Most of the time, food that gets stuck with gastric bypass patients is meat that has been well-chewed into a giant mush ball. I'm no longer surprised when the patient tells me it was just one bite, but when I perform a scope to fish it out, I find a big mush ball of meat.

Sometimes when a patient is out of the room, his or her family member or friend will tell me how often the patient is bringing food back up. This is common with my adopted patients, but I've never heard it about my patients. I hope this is an indication that our preoperative educational empowerment program is working.

If something gets "stuck", what should you do?

Most patients say waiting works. It will usually pass within two to five minutes. While waiting, getting up and walking around may help the food pass faster. Some Lap-Band websites mention Productive Burps or "PB's." This is where you belch the food particle back up, and it is usually accompanied by a slimy film. I think it is just a nice way of saying "vomiting without retching." There is less discussion about this with the sleeve or bypass.

I teach my patients never to let themselves get into this situation in the first place. You can do this by taking small bites, chewing thoroughly, taking your time, and stopping when you are satisfied. I believe this almost never happens with fresh fruits and vegetables, but occurs most often with meat, which is one of several reasons why I encourage my patients to move towards a pescatarian diet. However, this is anectdotal, as I'm not aware of any studies that have looked at this issue.

After the food piece has cleared, you must not eat another bite of this meal. Don't save it and try eating it for dinner—you're just not ready for it. At a minimum, back down to the next lowest food texture. For example, if chicken gave you trouble, then revert back to fish, which is easier to chew. If red meat was the culprit and it was a particularly bad episode, then I would even consider being on liquids for a while. Give your body two or three days before you try again. If it gets stuck a second time, avoid it all together and resign yourself to the fact that you might not be able to eat that food for a long time. The reason you need to back down to liquids or mushy foods is because the pouch will temporarily swell or become inflamed, like when you hit your thumb with a hammer. **Would you hit your swollen thumb again?** No, of course not. So don't eat again until that swelling goes down. There's no way to tell exactly how long that will take, because it depends on how bad the food was stuck, how recently you had surgery, and what type of surgery you had. I would encourage you to give it a couple of days. Start with liquids, work your way up to mushy foods and then soft vegetables over the course of a few days, not a few meals.

Also, don't mix up your food. One well-intentioned patient told me that rice got stuck. When he explained what he had eaten, he said he had made an Asian-style meal with thinly sliced beef, broccoli, and rice, and that when he ate the rice, it gave him trouble. I probed a bit further and he explained that he had placed all of the ingredients into a big bowl and mixed them together. I asked, "So you picked out one item at a time? You ate the broccoli, waited, then ate the beef, waited, then ate the rice and had trouble?" He realized his mistake and said, "No, I put a little of everything on my fork and ate it."

This is problematic for a couple of reasons. First, he doesn't know which food item was the culprit. Was it really the rice, like he thought? Or was it actually the broccoli or the meat? Because he mixed it all together, there is no way to be sure. Second, if he was able to take a little of everything on his fork, he took too big of a bite! This was probably a lapse back to his old habits. Old habits are hard to shake, but changing them is important to avoid this sort of problem.

Over-consumption of alcohol is another common cause of food getting stuck. Patients will have one too many drinks, get tipsy, forget their techniques, and take too big of a bite or not listen to their cues. They get stuck and have a food accident. This can be easily avoided if you do one simple thing: do not drink any alcohol until after you've eaten all that you are going to eat.

What should you NOT do when food is stuck?

If food is stuck, it is likely stuck in your esophagus, which is the long tube connecting your mouth to your stomach. Think of it like your kitchen sink drain. If something gets stuck, DO NOT DRINK WATER, hoping to force it down. Like your clogged sink, it will only back up and make your life miserable. Instead, stand up, walk around, and wait for it to pass. Then don't eat that food item again for at least several days.

What is the Second Rule of WLS Eating?

Fill your pouch with the most nutritious food you can most of the time.

Social Eating with the Gastric Sleeve

.

Social Eating with the Gastric Sleeve (Quiz)

What is the First Rule of Gastric Sleeve Eating?

Write down one social situation in which this rule applies.

After your gastric sleeve surgery, how will ordering food be different?

What about drinking before and with dinner?

What is the problem (or problems) with alcoholic drinks?

What is one strategy for keeping on track if you decide to splurge at an upcoming party?

Do you want to learn to cook, or re-learn to cook?

Remember, if you do what you've always done, you will get what you've always gotten. So when it comes to socializing, what is one thing that you will commit to changing?

Social Eating with the Gastric Sleeve (Answers)

What is the First Rule of Gastric Sleeve Eating?

Everybody all at once now: "Protein First!"

Write down one social situation in which this rule applies.

This is an important question to consider carefully. Many people can easily recite rules by memory and some claim to know everything that they are SUPPOSED to do, but few can actually implement those rules consistently. I don't think it is because they are incapable of understanding the rules, but rather that they've never been shown how to actually use them in real life. If you are to be a happy sleeve patient, you must understand how to make your sleeve work for you during social situations. I will provide several situations in which this rule applies. This list is in no way meant to be complete. Hopefully once you've mastered it, you can add your own examples and share them with other weight loss surgery colleagues.

I already mentioned how this rule applies at a restaurant and some strategies for sticking to it. Simply wait to eat anything until your main course arrives. Either do without the free salad (since most appetizer salads at restaurants are not healthy) or ask for it to be served with your entrée. Don't have anything from the bread basket. Pass on the chips and salsa. This is a good rule even for people who have not had weight loss surgery, but are struggling with their weight, because it is easy to consume several hundred calories before the main course even arrives.

At a party, this rule would mean that you should avoid the snacks and appetizers that circulate. Since this is very hard to do when you are hungry, try to eat before going to a party or an event that features a buffet. And what should you eat before going? Protein! Have a chicken breast sandwich or piece of fish. When you've already eaten, you can probably resist the appetizers or sample one small snack at the party and not be tempted to fill up on high-calorie treats. Another trick is to keep a glass (of sparkling water, for example) in your hand. That will keep you from feeling awkward while everyone else has a plate and also make it a difficult balancing act should you be tempted to sample something. And remember that with the sleeve, you should not eat near to the time you drink (see Question #4 below). Do not make the mistake of "saving" your calories for a party. Not only will you end up eating far more calories (and most likely empty calories) than you should, you will also be at risk of having food get stuck. That's definitely not something you want to have happen in a crowded room!

Of course, if people don't know why you suddenly are not eating much food, they may try to pressure you into eating more than you want or should. Whether at a restaurant, a business luncheon, or a family reunion, you can either tell them about your surgery or politely insist that you are trying to make healthier choices and that your restraint is in no way an insult!

After your gastric sleeve surgery, how will ordering food be different?

When I ask weight loss surgery patients this question, most say that they now order their meal from the appetizer portion of the menu, that they ask for half of their main course to be boxed up before it is even served, or that they just share some of their spouse's or friend's meal. While these are all great, there are two more things that I want my patients (and you) to understand about life after weight loss surgery.

It is ok to throw food away. You do not have to clean your plate. Forgive yourself for breaking this well-ingrained American familial law. After you have surgery, it should be impossible for you to consume all of the food on a typical plate in one sitting. I say "should" because there are ways around everything. Many of us were raised hearing that we could not go play until we'd cleaned our plate. Now, feel how liberating it is to leave some food behind and go do something else!

This is also true for times when you eat at restaurants. Let the waiter take away the food. Don't ask for a to-go box. I've seen people take the chips and salsa because "it would be a shame to let them go to waste—and besides, they're free." It might be free on the restaurant check, but if you keep eating these empty calorie foods, you'll pay for them in other ways. You'll pay with swollen ankles, heart failure, kidney failure, greasy skin, etc...and then, of course, the doctor's and pharmacist's bills!

You have to try different types of food. I often repeat the mantra, "If you do what you've always done, you will get what you've always gotten." Since you are trying to change your health, you must change your habits. This does not have to be a dreaded experience but can actually be fun! There is such a bountiful assortment and variety of food for us to experience in this country. But sadly, I can count on one hand what most of the people who seek my help eat on a day-to-day basis. They usually go to the same three or four restaurants and order the same three or four items. For me, this is just not an interesting way to eat.

We love food in our clinic, and we want our patients to learn to love food again, too! I often bring an unusual fruit or vegetable to my weekly educational groups. I start by passing it around the group and ask everyone to guess what it is. Most of the time, they don't know. When I tell them what it is, like a cherimoya, they'll ask me, "Dr. V., where did you get that fruit?" They are quite surprised when I tell them that I found it across the street at the local grocery store. Sometimes, I will bring in different herbs and vegetables for a few consecutive weeks; then on the third or fourth week, I'll bring in a dish I made with those ingredients for them to taste. For example, once I brought in eggplant, then tofu, then Thai basil. The last week, I brought one of my favorite Asian dishes, which highlights all three of those ingredients.

You, too, can do this! Spend some time researching things on the Internet and watching good cooking videos on YouTube. Visit different grocery stores or shop at a local farmer's market to load up on fresh produce. Ask the vendors for advice on selection and nuances in flavor. People love to help, if you will only give them the chance. **Do not pass up the opportunity to learn something new.** Pull yourself out of your eating and shopping rut and experience new flavors at least a couple of times a week. Why is this important? Not only will it provide your body with a vast array of important vitamins and minerals, but it will also change your relationship with food.

Food is not the enemy!

But rather it is a source of both nourishment and enjoyment.

What about drinking before and with dinner?

Most patients know the "Do Not Drink 30 Minutes Before or 30 Minutes After You Eat" rule, but most do not think about how this applies in social situations. First, let me explain the origin of this well-known rule. It was started by Dr. Paul O'Brien, one of the great Lap-Band forefathers from Australia. He told me that he used to tell his patients not to drink one hour before and one hour after eating! At the same time, he told his patients that it was good to drink a glass of red wine, because as we all know, wine is meant to be consumed with meals in order to complement the flavors of the food. Patients complained, however, that they were confused by these two guidelines: one said not to drink for two hours, and the other said to drink wine in order to augment the meal. So Dr. O'Brien compromised and created the 30-minute rule. As you can see, it is rather arbitrary, but it is grounded in good intentions.

The thinking behind this rule is that liquid will push food through your band faster and thus negate the purpose of the Lap-Band (or any weight loss procedure), which is to have real food sit in your pouch and create a sense of satiety. But I am not sure that this "rule" has ever been validated, although some patients swear by it. I will leave it up to your own personal experience to determine its efficacy, but if you prefer not to risk overeating, then just stick to the rule.

For me, it doesn't make much sense, since liquids should always go through your weight loss pouch (whether gastric bypass, gastric sleeve, or band) within a couple of minutes. If that is true, then the liquid you drink BEFORE dinner should not be sitting around, diluting your meal. Hopefully that liquid is water and not empty calories, like soda. But, as I said, some patients adhere to this rule with great results.

What is the problem (or problems) with alcoholic drinks?

As I've said earlier, a regular margarita can pack up to 600 calories. These are not good calories either, but rather empty ones that provide you with no nutrients. Calories aside, other pitfalls abound.

Many times in social situations where alcoholic beverages are served, less than ideal snacks are also being served. Take your average Super Bowl

Sunday, for example. Think about all of the tempting, deep-fried finger foods, hamburgers, chips, dips, candies, sweets, etc. All of these things can wreak havoc on anyone who is trying to make healthier choices. Alcohol lowers our inhibition, and we are far more likely to throw caution to the wind after a couple of beers. Most of us can recall a personal experience in which alcohol made us act a little more freely than usual. And when people around us are overindulging, it becomes even harder to resist. I am not suggesting that you will never have another alcoholic beverage again or never be able to attend another Super Bowl party. I am just stressing the importance of understanding the choices that you make, and if you prepare for the consequences that come with those choices, then you will be well on your way to successful long-term weight loss.

I've had sleeve patients report to me that they get intoxicated faster after the sleeve (one patient went from being able to consume seven or eight beers to feeling buzzed after just one and a half beers.) I'm not sure why this would occur with the sleeve, but patients don't seem to mind, and some actually think of it as a bonus side effect! They don't miss the extra calories and are still able to enjoy drinks from time to time.

What is one strategy for keeping on track if you decide to splurge at an upcoming party?

Note the question's construction – you *decide* to splurge. That's right, it's you're decision, because **you are in control.** Socializing is a part of everyday life. It is neither healthy nor realistic to think that the key to dieting success is to avoid all parties. Celebrations happen, and you should be able to take part in the festivities of graduations, anniversaries, holidays, weddings, reunions, bar mitzvahs, sweet sixteens—you name it. You just have to understand the choices you make regarding those occasions. I discuss this in the section titled "The 21 Days Exception."

Here is the key: if you are going to CHOOSE to splurge for that occasion, it is imperative that you make up for those extra calories, not the day before or two days before or even three days before, but the ENTIRE WEEK before! This is the guideline we give to our patients. I insist on this, not because I am a cruel despot, but because of the realistic rate of calorie expenditure versus the density of empty calories available at parties (more on this later). Trim back on portions, bump up your vegetable intake, and add a few minutes to your morning walk. You can easily find ways to cut a couple of hundred calories every day, and after five days or so you should feel free to enjoy the foods at the party. But making these choices ahead of time will also make that second slice of cake less tempting, because you will be more aware of what is in it. Be realistic about whether or not you will splurge; indulging should be a conscious decision and not a spur-of-the-moment impulse. Thinking through the potential pitfalls along your weight loss journey and planning for them will help you to stay on track, but it requires self-reflection and honesty.

Do you want to learn to cook, or re-learn to cook?

Why do I ask you (dare or challenge you) with a question that seems so simple at first glance? To put it simply, anything you prepare fresh from fresh ingredients is better than anything you buy at a restaurant or get from a can or a box or the freezer aisle—yes, even if that box or meal is labeled "Lean," "Sugar Free!" "Fat-Free," or "New and Improved." Take a moment and think about what has to go into these processed "food" items in order to give them a shelf-life of weeks, months, and even years, in some cases. Some shelf items will outlive me! Is that REAL FOOD? Is that what you really need to be putting into this one-and-only body of yours? **Why is it that we will put premium gas or high quality oil in our cars, but we give our bodies the cheapest and lowest quality fuel we can find?**

Most restaurants don't prepare their food on site. Their menu items are usually shipped to the restaurant in huge bags of processed and frozen products that are then assembled in the kitchen. This to me is not real food and definitely not real cooking. And you end up paying a lot more for it in the long run, in terms of your wallet or your health.

When I ask my patients what the biggest benefit of cooking is, they usually respond by saying that you can control the ingredients that go into the dish. You can use skim milk instead of heavy cream, for example. While this is true, it's not the biggest benefit.

> *The biggest benefit to cooking your own meals is that...you get to control your portion size.*

Portion size affects your caloric intake far more than ingredient choices, like substituting olive oil for a pat of butter. Using fresh ingredients is important, but it will not get you the same results as reducing portion size. When you cook your meals, you should prepare enough for you and your family to eat without having leftovers. That is my goal for my family when I cook. How do you do this? Buy just enough ingredients for each person's proper portion size. For example, when making green beans, I grab one handful for me, one handful for Melissa, and one small handful for our child, Kizzie. If you decide to have pasta, then just make enough for one serving for each person. This is much better than knowing you have the option of an "Endless Pasta Bowl." One serving of fettuccine Alfredo is bad enough, two is horrible, and endless is unthinkable.

Also, if you are cooking your meal, what are the chances you will be baking endless breadsticks, too? And an endless salad with heavy dressing? And a couple of endless sides? And what does the waiter always ask you right before she brings the check? "Can I tempt you with dessert?" What is the likelihood you will bake a three-layer chocolate fudge cake on a Tuesday night? Most people would not cook like this on an average Tuesday night, but there are a lot of restaurants that will offer this to you any day and almost any time of the week.

If you already know how to cook and currently prepare all of your meals, take time to re-evaluate the techniques you are using in the kitchen. It is not ok to think that you are being healthy if you serve steamed broccoli but then cover it with a thick cheese sauce or if bacon is your main ingredient. But for most of my patients who are cooks, their success or lack of it boils down to portion size and second helpings. Practice eating on a side plate and using a child spoon or fork, at least initially, until taking small bites becomes second nature. If you take small bites, you'll be forced to eat more slowly, which means you will feel full after consuming less food.

> *After you learn to master portion size, learn to use the best ingredients.*

Great chefs often talk about the importance of using the best ingredients, but a lot of people complain that the best ingredients are too expensive. I also faced this dilemma when I was starting out as a poor surgical resident. Here is how I handled the issue of cost. First, I started by spending a fair amount of money on staple items for the pantry, like good olive oil, organic rice wine vinegar, and Kosher salt that all last a long time. Then I moved on to purchasing small amounts of limited-shelf-life, quality ingredients for each meal — like organic vegetables, grains, and organic meats when available — but I only bought enough for one or two meals. This really kept prices down as I was learning how to master portion sizes. Yes, sometimes I would have to pay more per pound, but overall the amount I spent was less because I wasn't throwing out a lot of spoiled food and wasn't eating at restaurants often. I also learned complimentary recipes that use similar ingredients so that I could be sure to not waste any products. For example, if I bought snow peas, I'd cook tofu with snow peas that night and chicken, snow peas, and carrot stir-fry a couple of days later. Lastly, I learned recipes that repurposed any leftovers I might have. Tossing a bunch of items from the refrigerator into stir-fried noodles is a popular Asian method of using leftovers and aging produce, but making gumbo, stew, and soups serves the same purpose. If you use this method, then **cost should never be an excuse for not cooking healthily.**

Cooking is a great way to create lasting, meaningful memories with your family. Get your children involved in the process. This will not only teach them new skills, but also ingrain in them an appreciation for the nourishment we put in our bodies. Can't think of how you can do this? Here are a few tips.

- Have your children help you with prep work that is age-appropriate, like snapping green beans or rolling limes, washing salad leaves, or stirring. My daughter loves to use the salad spinner.
- Have them help you clean up. The tasks of transference and stacking that occur when they put things away develop critical motor skills. This also teaches them to be clean and orderly!
- Take them shopping at outdoor farmers markets to see all of the fresh ingredients and where they come from. A patient once told me she didn't realize that beans came from the ground. She had never put much thought into it, so she was quite surprised to see them growing from the ground in our patient gardens at my office. Perhaps you will discover a new fruit or vegetable together!
- Reconnect with Mother Earth by starting and growing an herb garden or a few vegetables. This is an invaluable opportunity to teach your kids

about nature and ecological cycles. My daughter has been digging for earthworms and playing with garden bugs with me since she was 18 months old. She has never been bitten, stung, or hurt by it. She is now curious about everything in this world, in all aspects of her everyday life, and I can't help but think that her curiosity was honed during "playtime" in the garden with Daddy.

Before you say, "I don't know anything about science", "I hate bugs", or "I can't___, can't___, can't___," ask yourself this question: "**What would I be willing to do if it meant that my child would avoid the same path of weight struggles that I've taken?**"

Besides, it could be fun to learn something new and have an excuse to get out a bit more. You don't have to do everything at once, but do try something!

Remember, if you do what you've always done, you will get what you've always gotten. So when it comes to socializing, what is one thing that you will commit to changing?

That was how I phrased the question in my first book. Now I think the question is more accurately stated as "If you do what you've always done, you'll get even less!" This is because the returns are so much worse these days—the foods are higher in calories, the nutrition is poorer, the portions are larger, the marketing is even more pervasive. I promise you will get much, much less if you keep doing what you've always done. This is one reason why losing weight is so much harder the older you get. Also, society's expectations are so much more extreme now, too. People demand so much more, expect so much more, want so much more from you that doing the same things the same way will have ever diminishing returns.

How do you correct this?

> *You must change what you have always done.*

There is no way to get around this. It's just like getting financially healthy: you've got to spend less than you earn. There's no way of getting around that if you want to grow wealthy. The same is true for losing weight—you must change what you've always done.

Don't wait; do it now! Write it down and commit to starting something new! Start with a small change. Here is a simple tip to making a change that you can stick with: Don't give something up but rather ADD something new. Add some walking, add some vegetables, add some quality family cooking time. The more you add, the less time and space you'll have for old, bad habits.

What is My Happy Weight?

What is My Happy Weight? (Quiz)

What does "Ideal BMI" mean? What does "Happy Weight?" mean? How are they different?

If you have already decided, then what is your Happy Weight?

How did you arrive at your number or goal for your Happy Weight?

Write down three things you can do to achieve your Happy Weight.

What is an activity other than social eating that you will do with friends/family?

Do you know of anyone who undermines your efforts to reach your Happy Weight? If so, what can you do to make this person more supportive?

What is one thing you will change right now to make yourself happier?

What is the Third Rule of Weight Loss Surgery?

What is My Happy Weight? (Answers)

What does "Ideal BMI" mean? What does "Happy Weight?" mean? How are they different?

It is not meaningful to say, "I am overweight because I weigh 250 pounds." There is a significant difference between a woman who is 5 feet tall and 250 pounds and a man who is 6 feet 2 inches tall, 250 pounds, and also happens to be a linebacker. BMI, or Body Mass Index, is a medical term that accounts for height and approximates a person's ideal body weight. An ideal BMI is considered to be between 19 and 25; anything higher than 25 is considered a signal of being overweight. It is not a perfect measure, but a good starting point. Most of you know your BMI already, but in case you don't, there are many free BMI calculators on the internet.

The BMI is by no means a perfect measure of health and fitness, but it provides a rough indication of the sorts of health problems a person may have. Why is it not perfect? There are other qualities that it does not take into account, such as :

Bone Frame. Some people have larger skeletal frames than others. You might have heard people say, "We are just big-boned." While there is a slight difference among various ethnic groups in the size of some major bones, I think that we tend to over-estimate its significance. I have also found that many patients have been incorrectly describing themselves this way for years.

Muscle-to-fat ratio. Lean muscle burns calories much more efficiently than fat does. Lean muscle provides the svelt look that our society has come to recognize as beautiful. When we are young and running around, we develop a certain amount of lean muscle, based on our activity level (think of dancers and soccer players), but as we get older or become more sedentary, we lose this lean muscle. Just sitting in a chair, if two people weigh the same, the lean person will burn more calories than the person with excess fat. Scientists now think that once your body creates a fat cell, it never goes away. When you lose weight, you deplete the fat that is stored in fat cells, but the fat cells themselves are still there, just waiting to receive fat again when you fall off your diet. In other words, you can lose muscle cells, but you can never lose fat cells. **So I tell my patients that their goal is not to lose weight, but to gain lean muscle!**

Age. The BMI does not ask how old you are. This is a big factor in our weight and health. As we age, we lose muscle mass, and guess what it's replaced with? That's right, FAT! If you take a 25-year-old woman with a BMI of 40 and fast forward her life until she turns into a 55-year-old woman with the same BMI, you will find that her body shape is very different, even though her BMI is the same. This is primarily due to the loss of her muscle mass and corresponding increase in fat. Her BMI of 40 at age 55 is much more detrimental to her health than the same BMI was at age 25 because of the relatively higher proportion of fat to muscle cells.

Gender. BMI does not take into account whether you're male or female. Typically, men can lose weight much faster and more easily than women. If you've ever gone on a diet with your husband (or wife, if you're a man), then you will know what I am talking about! This is most likely due to the fact that men typically have more lean muscle mass and are more physically active on a day-to-day basis.

Your Happy Weight, on the other hand, is the weight at which you are not struggling with your relationship with food. You look good, you feel good, and you have a fun social life. You're confident, you're active, and you're out there participating in life. This might be a BMI under 25, but it could also be a BMI over 25. It just depends on YOU, YOUR particular journey, and where YOU are at this point in YOUR life. I don't know where in your journey you are currently, but if you are contemplating starting your journey, trying to lose those "last 10 pounds," or regaining weight you had already lost, then stop reading this book right now. Spend a few minutes thinking about the following statement: **Everything you have in your life right now is a result of the choices you have made and are currently making.** If you are regaining weight after weight loss surgery, it is because of the food choices you are making. If you have lost a lot of weight and can't seem to drop those last 10 pounds, it could be because embarrassment is stopping you from finding a way to have plastic surgery to remove excess skin. If you can't seem to start your journey for a new, healthier life, it may be because the pain of your current situation is not great enough to compel you to act differently. Think honestly about what choices are keeping you in your current situation and which you are willing to change.

Your Happy Weight changes—especially after weight loss surgery—depending on what you want from your life and your health and more importantly on what you want to DO with your life. So think about your Happy Weight often.

If you have already decided, then what is your Happy Weight?

It's ok if you haven't decided on a Happy Weight, especially early in your weight loss journey. The important point is that you start thinking about your new life and what it will be like. Some of my patients don't pick a number. Instead, they set other measurable goals—like clothing size, medication change, or walking endurance. For example, my early post-op patients might say, "I want to fit into a single digit dress size," "I want to get off my blood pressure medications," or "I want to be able to walk to do my grocery shopping." These are great goals to set!

How did you arrive at your number or goal for your Happy Weight?

This is a very important question. If you left this question blank, go back and answer it now. You have to understand the motivations behind the decisions you make. What drove you to give the answer you gave? How you derived your Happy Weight is just as important as the actual Happy Weight itself. If you write down that it's what you read some Hollywood actor weighs, then you might need to think more about what you would be happy with. A motivation that stems from your personal desires will help carry you through the difficult times, but one that stems from some Hollywood ideal can be discouraging and unrealistic.

When patients say something like, "I want to weigh 185 pounds," I ask, "How did you arrive at that number?" Then they will usually say, "Well, that's how much I weighed when I was a high school senior and was on the football team."—or cheerleader in college, or whatever. It is important that you realize, however, that your body has changed, so even if you reach that number, you will probably not look the same way you did back then. Your lean muscle mass is different. The elasticity of your skin will be different. If you're a smoker, then those years of smoking will have an effect on the color and texture of your face. If you now have three kids or are starting your own business, then that stress will show up in the bags under your eyes. Set new goals based on your life now. You probably won't be a high school football star again, but you could have fun kicking the ball around with an office team or with your kids.

Write down three things you can do to achieve your Happy Weight.

This should be easy. There are many resources available to help you with this one. Try books, the Internet, e-newsletters, etc. The web site, www.WLSchannel.com, is the first Internet channel completely devoted to the care of weight loss surgery patients. VerticalSleeveTalk.com is an online social site where you can meet and blog with other sleeve patients. There are lots of weight loss surgery groups on Facebook, including my own. This is just a small sampling of the many resources out there to help get you started and keep you motivated.

Here are a few ideas about how to achieve your Happy Weight:

- **Enlist support from your closest friends and family.** Support is everything in weight loss, because social interactions are key to everyday happiness. The people you spend your time with can help you achieve your goals, or they can lure you back into old habits. Getting them on board with your new lifestyle is essential to your success.

- **Add extra, simple activity at work.** Instead of calling your co-worker, walk down the hall to deliver the message; instead of rolling in the chair, get up and walk. Stand while talking on the phone. Offer to pick up forms from another building. Without adding much time or effort, you can increase your calorie expenditure by at least 100 calories a day. Many studies have shown that people who constantly "fidget" (tapping their foot or shifting in their chairs) also tend to weigh less. Small bits of movement add up.

- **Cut down on alcohol consumption.** If you are used to regular drinks, cutting them out entirely can be difficult; instead, cut back a little more each week. Alcohol not only has a lot of calories in itself, but it also encourages us to make poor choices.

- **Learn to cook real food or change how you cook.** Remember, anything you cook from real ingredients is better than anything you buy already prepared, even if it says "Weight Watchers" on the box.

- **Start an easy and convenient exercise routine.** Convenience is key because it reduces the number of excuses you can come up with to avoid it!

- **Change your driving routine** to avoid old temptations like donut shops and fast food restaurants. I had a patient who used to stop at McDonald's to get an order of fries every day on the way home from work. If this sounds like you, then don't drive near the McDonald's. If you're feeling tired or stressed, it will be hard to resist your old routine.

- **Be happy.** If you are enjoying your life and the people with whom you are spending your time, you will achieve your goals more easily. In fact, this is the main message we try to deliver to our patients:

Seek Happinesess, not Thinness.

A technique that I find successful for anything you want in life, not just weight loss, is to write down a BIG goal, set a date for achieving that goal, and then break it down into smaller increments. Let's say you are 100 pounds overweight and want to lose them in 12 months. That breaks down to only 8.3 pounds a month, about two pounds a week, or 0.3 lbs a day! Small choices every day can get you to these smaller goals: pass on the cheesecake at lunch, drink water instead of Mountain Dews, choose grilled fish instead of fattening chicken Alfredo, or eat a banana for breakfast instead of Pop Tarts. But the KEY is that you've got to do this for a year, not just one day. The goal you set was for 12 MONTHS, not 12 DAYS! You are where you are now because of a few years (maybe a lifetime) of bad habits, so I'm always perplexed when people give up on their new healthy lifestyle after a few weeks.

Success in anything relies more on perseverence than on anything else.

Thomas Edison said, "Success is 10% inspiration and 90% perspiration." So don't quit!

What is an activity other than social eating that you will do with friends/family?

Social gatherings are an integral part of life, but why do we make them all center on food? This world has so much else for us to experience. If you live in the city, your non-food options are almost limitless. Try visiting museums, zoos, planetariums, historical sites, old homes, monuments, etc. Go see plays or go to book readings. Call your local Chamber of Commerce if you lack ideas. Join groups with similar interests. There are walking groups, fitness groups, hiking groups, museum groups, all sorts of groups! You can find such groups on websites like www.meetup.com. There are community classes in watercolor, literature, country dancing, movie appreciation, gardening, almost anything you could possibly want to learn. If you don't live in the city, don't be discouraged. There are many of the same opportunities in small towns—you just have to look for them or start them yourself. And you probably have more open space for playing Frisbee or birdwatching.

A news report I heard on radio suggested that the root cause of obesity in America is our loss of connection to nature. I think there might be some truth to this. Plan outdoor games, kick the ball around, take a walk around the neighborhood after dinner, organize a family softball/football tournament, or try fishing or hiking trips. Plant a family garden and make it a criterion to use something from the garden if anyone wants to have a family get-together where food is involved. These are just some tips, but feel free to find your own and share them with me on my Facebook page.

Do you know of anyone who undermines your efforts to reach your Happy Weight? If so, what can you do to make this person more supportive?

It is important to know who your support people are and how to communicate your needs to them, so take this question very seriously. This can be scary, suggesting that you might have to acknowledge that someone near and dear to you might be subconsciously (or even consciously) undermining your weight loss efforts. Count yourself lucky if you can only think of one person. Many of my patients have multiple offenders.

You've got to take an honest account of those closest to you. Remember the old saying, "Actions speak louder than words." So despite what these people might say, it is important to determine whether or not their actions are consistent with their words. If someone says he is happy to see you trying to become healthier but then brings home your favorite dessert and eats it in front of you, he is not supporting your efforts!

Also determine whether anything you are doing contributes to this person's behavior. Are you empowering him to behave this way? If you want him to be more supportive, you have to tell him what you expect from him, what type of support you need, what questions to ask or not to ask, what kind words or critical words are helpful, etc. Deep down, this person loves you and wants you to succeed, but you have to let him know how to support you because no one can read your mind.

And if you determine that this person doesn't really love you or want to see you succeed, then you've got to decide how important it is to keep him in your life. That is why this question is so scary.

> *You are the average of your five closest relationships.*

If your five closest friends are overweight, chances are you, too, will be overweight. If they are always on a diet, you will probably also be on a diet. If your five closest relationships are spending more than they earn, can't seem to save money, live paycheck to paycheck, then chances are you, too, are doing the same—even if you earn more money than they do or have a "better job." If your five closest relationships have been divorced, struggle to find marital happiness, or have a lot of drama at home, then chances are you will, too. It's ok if you want to keep your current relationships as they are, but I will tell you, you've got to go out and seek better people to be your role models and exert influence over you.

What is one thing you will change right now to make yourself happier?

Ask yourself, "What will make me really happy?" It can be as complex as "Find a new job that I really love" or something as simple as "Be able to walk without my knees hurting." This is a Call To Action! Don't just think about it. Do it! Haven't you waited long enough? Aren't you tired of sitting on the sidelines, watching as life passes by you? Say these three simple words:

ENOUGH IS ENOUGH

What is the Third Rule of Weight Loss Surgery?

Kizzie's Rule: You can eat all the fresh fruits and vegetables you want, any time you want, as much as you want.

Refocus Your Focus

Refocus Your Focus (Quiz)

What was your eating pattern like prior to weight loss surgery?

What were your familial relationships like prior to your weight loss surgery?

What was work like prior to your weight loss surgery?

How did you spend your weekends prior to weight loss surgery?

How did you spend your family time? Name one activity you did together.

Name one charity for which you would like to volunteer and why.

Write the first sentence of your journal entry for today.

Do you keep a food diary?

Name one thing that is different in your life since your surgery.

What is one thing about your life that you will change right now?

Refocus Your Focus (Answers)

What was your eating pattern like prior to weight loss surgery?

Be honest. That is the key to this question. It is important to face the behaviors that got us to where we are because that is the only way we can change them. Sometimes our memories fail us. Sometimes we can't face the truth of our bad behaviors and the choices we've made in the past, so we find other reasons for our failures. Let me tell you, you're not alone. So that you might find some courage, here are some things my patients have told me:

- Regularly eating an entire half-gallon of ice cream in one sitting during stressful times, which in her mind meant nightly.
- Eating out seven days a week for all meals, just because.
- Going through the drive-thru at midnight on the way home from a night shift.
- Drinking 10 Diet Cokes® a day (remember that diet soda consumption is linked to obesity, even if the sodas themselves have zero calories).
- Eating an entire vat of gumbo.
- Hiding candy bars around the house, so her family couldn't find them.
- Buying a separate large pizza and eating it in the car before bringing a pizza home for her family's dinner.
- Waking up and eating lemon pie at 2 a.m.
- Making at least six trips a day for a Starbucks "skinny" latte.
- Despite eating multiple servings at a Chinese buffet, taking a to-go box, then eating it later that evening.

Remember, it is our SMALL EVERYDAY CHOICES that lead to success in life. So consider some of the good choices you may have been making, like eating fresh fruit every day, testing out new recipes, choosing water instead of sweet tea, or not allowing chips in the house. If you're reading this book, you are aware that you've made bad choices, but I'm sure you've also made some smart decisions. Just as important as recognizing what we need to change is reinforcing what we've been doing that is healthy.

What were your familial relationships like prior to your weight loss surgery?

Here are some questions for you to ponder:

- What role has family played in your current weight struggles? How far back can you trace this influence?
- Were you the "chubby child" or were you the "thin one?"
- What were your parents' attitudes about food and family dinners?
- What were your parents' attitudes about your physical appearance? How did this affect your body image?
- What is your fondest memory involving your family? Does it involve food?

Spend some time really thinking about these questions. You might be surprised with some of the answers you come up with. Most of the time, your memories won't involve food, and even if food is in the picture it plays a distant second role to the people. When you reflect on these good memories, hopefully you will realize that it is the FAMILY that is important and not the FOOD. Recognizing the role that family plays in your weight, however, can also help you to be proactive. Are you getting together with family for dinner, and everyone assumes you will take a second helping? Well, announce your plan beforehand and enlist their help in sticking to it. Have you always felt that your role in your family as the bigger sibling was a self-fulfilling prophecy? Well, tell your family that you don't like that role and want to change it.

> *Don't feel that you are stuck in a family dynamic over which you have no control.*

Take control and make those changes that will help you achieve success.

What was work like prior to your weight loss surgery?

Face it. We spend anywhere from 8 to 16 hours a day at work, maybe more, so work plays a really big role in our weight loss efforts. Once during residency, I spent 40 hours straight working at the hospital. This is the average number of work hours for an American for the entire week! And the typical food at a hospital is not very healthy, so I understand the challenges that our jobs may cause for our good health. Many people depend on regular paychecks to pay for their living expenses, but if your work environment is detrimental to your health, then you have to ask yourself if it is worth it. Or is there something else you could be doing, whether at your current job or a different one, to make your work environment healthier? Many corporations now have incentives for their employees to lose weight and stay healthier. Ask yourself, why haven't I participated in my employer's health program? Should I start a lunchtime walking group? Why don't I know where the stairs are located? What lunch options are there other than our usual fast food or buffet places? Is there a well-intentioned co-worker who brings donuts every Monday? Perhaps the baked goods could stay in a less-convenient place in the building. If you spend this much time at work, shouldn't you take steps to make it more health-friendly? And if you don't take a stand, then who will?

I have one patient, who worked as a dispatcher for first responders at the local 911 call center. When I first met her, even before she told me directly, I could sense that her job contributed to a lot of her weight problems. She said that her work fielding phone calls from people involved in car accidents, homes on fire, or major crimes like burglaries-in-progress, was "extremely stressful." And she often took the stress of those phone calls home with her. To make matters worse, the job's conditions also affected everybody's attitudes, so she didn't even like her coworkers much. Instead of being a supportive family unit, the staff bickered a lot. She responded to this stress with eating comfort foods at work and after she returned home. I knew if she didn't change her work environment somehow that her chances for success were greatly reduced. You can imagine my smile when she came to group one week and announced that she had gotten a new job! Her face was lit up like Christmas morning. And yes, she has been very successful with her weight loss goals and is much happier with her life goals, too!

How did you spend your weekends prior to weight loss surgery?

Our "free time" is just that—free time. But how do you spend it? Do you waste it away by sleeping in until noon, then wonder why you can't sleep at night and why you feel sluggish come Monday morning? Or do you wake up before sunrise in order to finish all of the "chores" that you have to get done or promised others you'd get done? Either way, ask yourself:

> *Am I really making my life the one I want to live?*

Or are you letting life pass you by? Are you willing to change this? On most weekends I'm involved with family, patient, or professional activities, yet I leave the weekend often feeling that I could have accomplished more. Even though it's Super Bowl Sunday, I'm still taking the time to type this, but I know that tomorrow, I'll wish I'd written a little bit more, planted another packet of seeds, read another chapter of a good book, and taken my daughter to the art museum. But I guess this is better than feeling like I haven't accomplished anything at all. An accomplishment to me doesn't mean getting the laundry done, but rather developing my next "Big Idea," going with patients and staff to participate in a 5K walk, planting our family garden with my daughter. These are things I can't always do on weeknights, and they make my weekend satisfying and memorable.

When they are asked, "What is your most valuable resource?" most people will respond with something like money, intelligence, or persistence. But the real answer is time.

> *Your most valuable resource is TIME.*

And we waste it every day. We all, whether a janitor or President of the United States, have only 24 hours in a day. Make a commitment now to not waste it. Turn off the television. Hang up the phone. Give up Farmville, Candy Crush, or online gaming. Do something productive that will get you to your goals. Today. Right now. Or this time next year, you'll be in exactly the same place—or maybe someplace even a little less satisfying.

How did you spend your family time? Name one activity you did together.

The important point is to realize that it is the FAMILY INTERACTION that is important. Did you spend your time making lasting memories or were you too busy in the kitchen, shuttling kids around, or shopping for more shoes to notice that you had missed out on those opportunities to make memories?

What will you do differently moving forward? Many wonderful family memories involve doing something together, just family. When you ask adults what they remember about their childhoods, most will not recall the exact activities or particular details about events, but rather just whether or not their parents were present—"They always came to my swim meets", "I wish my mom spent more time with us in the living room and less time in the kitchen", "I remember the day my dad took me to work with him." Make those same memories with the people around you now, the important ones that you consider your real family.

Name one charity for which you would like to volunteer and why.

I believe in charity work. In the past, I have partnered my practice with many charities. My patients, staff, and our families participate in fundraisers and charity walks regularly. In Houston, my two main partnerships were with the Snowdrop Foundation, which cares for children with cancer, and the Wounded Warrior Project, an international organization that helps American veterans who were wounded on the battlefield. I was on the board of D'Feet Breast Cancer, an organization that provides free mammograms and breast cancer care for impoverished women. My office and patients also volunteered for the Galveston Bay Foundation in trash cleanups and grass plantings. But why do I point this out?

I believe that it is critically important for your long-term weight maintenance to see the world from a broader perspective. Many people who struggle with their weight often become overwhelmingly self-focused. They may be filled with self-doubt and grow socially isolated. They may put themselves down or allow others to put them down, and the negative feelings this causes reinforces their poor habits. These poor habits, in turn, exacerbate the situation, and it becomes very difficult for them to see beyond their own weight struggles. It can be tough to pull yourself out of this cycle, but it is key to your success. Often it can be achieved by forming meaningful connections with others and seeing the difficult challenges that others face and overcome.

Thinking about the bigger picture will help put your weight struggles into perspective. When you meet a child who beat cancer or see an amputated war veteran helping with the table arrangements, you will think to yourself,

"Gee, maybe I don't have it so bad after all..." Then hopefully, you will start counting your blessings, rather than your shortcomings, and thinking momentum-building, positive thoughts rather than energy-sucking, negative ones. Once your weight loss struggles do not appear insurmountable, you'll see all the ways that you can empower yourself to become healthier and more vibrant. Don't say that you don't have time. Nobody will tell you there's something more important for you to do than serve meals in a soup kitchen for two hours or make crafts with kids in the hospital. Don't say that you can't because you have small children. My daughter loved "helping" to plant marsh grasses when she was one, two, and three years old, and some friends of ours foster small animals as they recover from injuries before they can be adopted. Don't say you can't because you have no energy. These sorts of activities will GIVE you energy, not sap it from you. Whatever the excuse, there's a way around it.

I believe deeply that donating your time and energy to a charity will help you to break free from that sense of isolation and fill your downtrodden spirit with renewed life and vigor! I honestly believe in that old saying:

> *Whatever you give, you will receive back ten-fold.*

I have already seen it in my own life. I immigrated to the United States as a little boy with my father. We spent months in a refugee camp in Thailand, and then a church sponsored us to come to America. We got off the plane in Houston with nothing but the clothes on our backs. We didn't even have a place to go. It was only through the generosity of the local government that we survived the night and through the generosity of a local church that we were able to set down roots. We lived in a closet for six months. I've gotten to where I am today in my life, every step along the way, largely through the generosity of others, and I have not forgotten this. Years later, when I was in college at Rice University, I found the papers that were given to me when I entered the Airport Authority. On those papers, the address of the people who had "sponsored" me was listed, and as it turned out, they lived on the same street where I currently was living! What were the odds? But they had moved away, so I never got to meet that family whose simple act of generosity changed my life forever. Isn't life funny that way?

What organization are you willing to give your time to? Whose life could you change? Money is always nice, but I've come to learn that most of these organizations just need your time. This is a win-win situation. They need your time, you've got time to give, and at the very least, you will get out of the house and get some physical activity. If you feel you don't have time, make it into a family activity or find something you can do during the lunch hour. There are so many organizations that need you, and there is certainly one that will spark your interest and fit into the amount of time you have to give. Don't let this opportunity pass you by; at the end of the day, you can feel that you have made the world a little better.

Write the first sentence of your journal entry for today.

This isn't the "Dear Diary" activity of adolescent girls, so don't be embarrassed. It is important to keep a journal. Write down what you did, how you were feeling when you did it, and why you think you did it. Your journal is the place where you can write down your thoughts and emotions and not worry about being judged. I carry a bound journal with me almost everywhere I go and use it to jot down ideas. I've learned not to trust my memory! I've found that I will quickly forget my ideas if I don't write them down. When I first started taking my journal into meetings with me, I used to be self-conscious about what others were thinking, but now I don't worry about it. Hospital administration has just gotten used to seeing me write in my journal now.

A simple spiral notebook will do just fine, but in today's world, you can do this online. You can blog online, you can post online, you can join groups online. The important thing is that you write, because writing may help you to understand the motivations that have led to your weight struggles and provide insight into how you can overcome them.

I teach my patients to use their Facebook status postings as a type of journal. I encourage them to scroll back through their updates and see the topics they chose to air "out there." Were they negative and petty or positive and uplifting? Did they offer insight or add to the constant complaining of the world? Are the postings nothing more than pictures of baked goods or cheesy casseroles, accompanied by phrases like, "This is to die for!"? This gives key insight into what their minds are focused on. I also tell my patients to review what status updates are showing up on their Facebook page. Are their "friends" posting a lot of negative statements? What does that say about whom they choose to have as friends? Facebook follows your likes and comments, so its algorithm teaches it which updates to show you. If it is showing you mostly negative updates, then it is demonstrating your preferences for these negative influences.

Facebook is the ultimate mirror of our social lives. Do you like what you are seeing in that mirror? If not, then you must change it.

Do you keep a food diary?

A weight loss surgeon from Arizona named Dr. Terry Simpson once gave a questionnaire to those patients who had lost greater than 90% of their excess weight. This questionnaire was hoping to find what these patients were doing differently from other, less successful patients. The survey found that these highly successful patients were doing one simple thing that the other group was not: they kept food diaries. While keeping a food diary might seem onerous to some, aren't the benefits worth it? A lot of patients willingly pay tens of thousands of dollars in cash for their surgeries but won't pay $1 for a food log. What would you be willing to pay to help you achieve that goal you are after? Would you pay $20 for a professionally bound food and exercise diary? How about paying $0.99 for a simple spiral notebook? Better than that, there are many online food diaries that will help you track your caloric intake for free. They can help you determine just how many calories are in a chicken breast or an ear of corn. Just write down everything you eat and seek out sites that help you gauge their nutritional value. You might like to try these online resources, but there are countless others as well:

a.   FitDay.com—This free, online resource gives you access to a weight loss journal, daily calorie counts, and nutritional information on thousands of foods.

b.   www.bodybugg.com—This is a small device that you wear on your arm that helps measure your daily caloric intake and expenditure.

c.   FoodFit.com—This site provides free expert information on healthy eating, healthy cooking, and fitness.

A food diary will help you track your eating habits. More importantly, if done correctly, it will help you find patterns in your thought processes that lead to food choices. Every time you meet with your clinic's dietitian, you should be prepared to show her your food diary. Would you ever meet with your accountant, but not give him a spreadsheet of your spending? If you are struggling with your weight, the first thing your clinic will tell you to do is to start keeping a food diary.

Name one thing that is different in your life since your surgery.

Give yourself some credit. Most people don't like to talk about their accomplishments because they feel it is akin to bragging, but that is not the case when it comes to taking your health into your own hands. Reflect on everything you've accomplished so far. Use this opportunity to set milestones in your weight loss journey, and I'm not just talking about the number on the scale, or the smaller clothing size, or the changes in your medication. Those are all good measures. But I think it is probably more important to acknowledge the other positive changes in your life. Are you a better mother because you have more energy to play with your children? Are you a better employee because you have more focus at work? Are you a better spouse because you are more emotionally available? Are you a better son or daughter because you help your family around the house and yard? Are you a better humanitarian because you donate your time to charities?

If you can't think of anything, don't be embarrassed. Ask someone you love! They will give you an honest answer. That is why it is important to have a few close relationships—they become the measuring gauge for how we are doing with our lives. And keep striving to do more, to grow into a better and better person.

What is one thing about your life that you will change right now?

It can be a big dream or a small step, but regardless of the immensity of the change, just go do it! Commit to it now. Whether your surgery took place last month, last year, or in the last decade, it was just the start of the journey. Now it is time to go live the rest of your life!

If you decide to make a change, I would strongly encourage you to

MAKE A BIG CHANGE!

Why not? Why continue to live timidly? Why take baby steps when you can make leaps and bounds?

It occurred to me one day, in the history of the world, there has never been anyone like me on this planet, and after I die, there will never be another person like me. We are all unique, each and every one of us. Go make a difference. Be noticed. Leave a mark. Set an example. Be an inspiration to others. You can do this. You matter. You've got something special in you because there has been and will ever be only one you.

The Maintenance Period – The Truth About Hunger

The Maintenance Period—The Truth About Hunger

Getting the gastric sleeve surgery is such an exciting step. You were likely highly motivated right after your surgery to be a healthier eater and more active person. The pounds probably dropped off quickly in those first weeks, and you were excited to be able to fit into smaller sizes. (It is not uncommon for my gastric sleeve patients, who follow my program closely, to lose 100 pounds within a six month time period.) Coworkers, friends, and family were all impressed with the changes they saw and regularly complimented your new lifestyle. All of this positive attention gave you not only a morale boost, but also constant reinforcement. Sometimes, it may have been hard learning how to eat, what to eat, and when to eat, but overall, it was pretty easy to lose weight. You ate a small amount of food and felt full.

Now the surgery is in the distant past. The small amount of food is not as satisfying or doesn't seem to hold you over as long. Your number one enemy, The Hunger, seems to be back on your doorstep more frequently and hangs around longer. Everyone has gotten used to the New You and nobody comments on how great you look, except occasionally when you bump into an old acquaintance. Walking way across the parking lot to your car and taking the stairs do not make you sweat like they used to, and remembering what Dr. Vuong said, you now feel even more pressure to include some real exercise into your day. But who has time to go to the gym these days? You have deadlines at work, increasing family obligations, fun social activities planned, and a lot else going on. You need to focus on so many aspects of your life right now that cooking a fresh meal takes a backseat to other items on your long list of things to do. And did I mention how hungry you are? Since you've shifted away from making your "new" lifestyle your number one priority, your weight loss probably has slowed or stopped. Perhaps you even put a few pounds back on. Hopefully, you haven't put most or all of it back on.

Patients have many reasons why the pounds are coming back, but the one I hear and read about the most on blogs is Hunger. "I'm getting hungry again! Oh, no! What do I do?!"

The Truth About Hunger

I have many preoperative patients say to me, "Dr. Vuong, I don't want to be hungry anymore." They are always surprised when I tell them that it is natural to be hungry. It is unnatural to be full. I, too, get hungry. And I know a lot about hunger. I spent six months in a refugee camp in Thailand as a young child. Most people who meet me don't realize this because even though I am Asian, I don't speak English with an accent. (Unless of course, that is, you count my slight Texas twang.) They just assume I was born in America. My father and I were some of the "boat people" you might have heard about after the Vietnam War ended. My father made a daring escape with me in his arms one dark night in a little boat full of people. We ended up coming ashore to a refugee camp in Thailand, where there were lots of refugees. Lots of skinny, dark-haired refugees. And very little food. So I am no stranger to hunger.

Whenever I get hungry, I eat. Hunger pangs are my body's way of telling me that it needs nourishment. I appreciate that simple luxury now—the gift of knowing that if I am hungry, I can easily find food. There is a reason why Thanksgiving only comes around once a year. It is unnatural to feel "stuffed." Problem is most Americans want it to be Thanksgiving at every meal. They want to feel full every time they eat and to never be hungry between meals. This is just not realistic. It is not how our bodies have evolved.

Unfortunately, the field of bariatrics has convinced many Americans that weight loss surgery will miraculously eliminate one's sensation of hunger and that one will feel full between meals. In my experience, I have found that this is just not true. I am very happy if my patients eat until they are satisfied at mealtime and are able to resist snacking between meals. This is because most snacks in America are not good for you. Snacking for Americans often means something "quick and easy." And when it comes to your health, "quick and easy" usually is not healthy for you. Snacks are conveniently located down the hallway at the nearest vending machine. Sometimes, they are not even that far away. Sometimes, they are right in our own desk drawers or on the countertop. We have to learn to resist this snacking temptation. Snacking, for the most part, is an American invention. The rest of the world typically does not snack. Even if you are a diabetic, I strongly recommend that you minimize your snacking. Because the truth about hunger is this:

> *In order to lose weight, you must reduce your caloric intake; in order to reduce your caloric intake, you must allow yourself to become hungry.*

As you lose weight and become more active, your body will need more energy to keep it going. It will need better fuel than what it has gotten in the past. The body's fuel gauge for energy is REAL HUNGER.

I teach my patients to try and figure out whether they are really hungry or whether they are just feeling psychological hunger. Real hunger manifests itself with measurable physical changes—decreased blood sugar, weakness, sweating, jitteriness, dizziness, etc. Psychological hunger does not come with these physical changes (even though your stomach may still rumble), but rather is triggered by the thought, sight, or familiar smell of food. This is often situational. For example, you might develop cravings when a food commercial comes on while you're watching your favorite TV show or you walk by a cookie stand. So, if you feel hungry, make sure it is really hunger that you are feeling. Drinking a big glass of water usually helps. Assess whether it is an appropriate time to be hungry and verify that you are not in a situation that could trigger psychological hunger. If you put yourself in a different situation—you turn off the TV and go outside or you move away from the smells of baking, for example—you might find that you're not "hungry" a few minutes later.

A lot of my patients think they are eating too much (maybe this is because I have them practice eating from a little saucer full of food). After reviewing their meals, I am happy to point out to most of my patients that they are actually eating the right amount of food! It is just more than what they THOUGHT they should eat. Sometimes, I point out that they should increase the texture of what they eat. Maybe they are scared to move away from mushy tuna fish salad and have been avoiding chicken or meat for fear that it would get stuck. The Texture Scale is useful in these situations. "A meal" is something very different for a weight loss surgery patient. Sometimes, this is very hard for patients to understand or recognize.

Here is a not-too-uncommon scenario from a gastric band patient. A week after her first adjustment, she complained that she was hungry and thought the adjustment "didn't work", even though we explain to our patients that the average number of adjustments the first year is four or five and can vary between two and ten—or even more! After talking with her, it became apparent that she was stressed out about something. Turns out, it was the one-year anniversary of her father's passing. Eventually, she said, "I don't even know why I am eating—I'm not even hungry when I do it..." which was the opposite of her original complaint. We hugged really hard, and I encouraged her to come to support group. I haven't had this scenario as much with my gastric sleeve patients. I find that their hunger drive is much more suppressed, at least initially.

I tell my patients that whenever they get hungry, the first thing they should do is drink a big glass of water and then wait 10 minutes. After 10 minutes, if they are still hungry, then they can eat, if it is an appropriate time. More often than not, they will find that this "hunger" is not true hunger at all, but rather that it is more closely related to some emotion or condition, such as boredom, sadness, or loneliness. So, if you want to be successful in your weight loss journey, you must reevaluate your perception of hunger. You must realize that hunger is not the enemy. It is a natural part of being you. And in order to be successful you must embrace all aspects of you. So remember:

> *It is natural to be hungry; it is unnatural to be full.*

If you experience weight gain or weight plateau or if you want to avoid this scenario, then now is the time to read this next section.

When asked what it is that I do for a living, most people would answer that I am a weight loss surgeon. I say, "No, I am a motivator of people." My number one job is to constantly motivate those around me, and that includes you reading this book. My background as a hungry but happy child in a refugee camp gives me a slightly different insight into food, health, and hunger that I don't think is taught very well in medical school. You need motivation to stick to your healthy choices and overcome your weight-loss "plateau." You can reach your happy weight, walk in a local 5K, get through the holidays without putting on pounds, or reach any of your other goals. You have the answers to your struggles, the trick is unlocking them. The aim of this section is to give you that motivational boost, to provide you with simple tips to get back on track, and to encourage you always to make your own health a priority.

Start by thinking about all you have accomplished since your gastric sleeve surgery, both in terms of your health and the rest of your life. Give yourself proper credit for these accomplishments. And then resolve to accomplish even more.

The Weight Loss Plateau

The Weight Loss "Plateau" (Quiz)

One of the greatest motivators to stick with your weight loss program is seeing the pounds drop off. When you hit the dreaded "Plateau" and your weight loss levels off, you might get discouraged. Rather than doubt yourself or your program, take the time to understand what triggers a plateau and how to move past it.

Are you eating enough protein? How many grams of protein a day should you eat?

Could it be that you are drinking your daily calories? List any drinks you are consuming that contain calories and how frequently. What is wrong with diet drinks?

Could it be that you are not drinking enough water? How much water are you drinking a day? How much water should you be drinking a day?

Could it be that you are not eating enough? How many times a day should you eat after gastric sleeve surgery?

What is the minimum number of calories you should consume to avoid metabolic slowdown? How can you combat a slow metabolism?

Are you consuming empty calories (calories without any nutritious value)? Any at all? Write down everything you have eaten since breakfast yesterday morning and evaluate your choices.

The Weight Loss "Plateau" (Answers)

One of the greatest motivators to stick with your weight loss program is seeing the pounds drop off. When you hit the dreaded "Plateau" and your weight loss levels off, you might get discouraged. Rather than doubt yourself or your program, take the time to understand what triggers a plateau and how to move past it.

Are you eating enough protein? How many grams of protein a day should you eat?

Remember the First Rule of WLS Eating? "Yes, Dr. Vuong. Protein First." Great! But how much is enough? The accepted recommendation is 50 to 60 grams of protein per day for the average person, but I know of some bariatric programs that are pushing 80 or 90 grams of protein a day on their weight loss surgery patients. I think this is really too much. I suggest that my patients comfortably eat about 45 to 55 grams of protein a day, with much of that coming from leaner sources (see Appendix D). The exact number depends on the size of the patient. I cannot tell a 5-foot-tall grandmother to eat the same amount of protein as a 6'2" college student.

"Yes, I know the number of grams, but how much should I EAT?" you ask.

Putting the knowledge into practice is a struggle in itself. As a guideline, I recommend the "1-2-3 Rule for Protein." You should eat:

1 ounce of protein for breakfast,

2 ounces for lunch, and

3 ounces for dinner.

Remember one ounce of meat = about seven grams of protein. I'll get to the math of the 1-2-3 Rule later. Ok, now how much is an ounce, you ask? A good approximation is that a deck of cards is about the size of three ounces of protein. One of those slim smart phones is about three ounces. To get two ounces, just approximate a portion size about two-thirds the size of a deck of cards! Another easy trick is to remember that one boiled egg is about one ounce of protein. That should make breakfast a cinch!

Here's an example of the 1-2-3 Rule in action:

Breakfast: Big glass of water, coffee, boiled egg, small banana = About 7 grams of protein

Lunch: Big glass of water, super-large mixed salad with raw veggies and 2 ounces of chicken on it = About 14 grams of protein

Dinner: Big glass of water, veggies, grilled, 3-ounce fish filet on a bed of couscous = 21 grams of protein.

7+14+21 = 42 grams of protein for the day.

"But Dr. Vuong, that's not enough protein!" you shout.

You would be correct IF all you did was count "animal" sources of protein. Remember that veggies and whole grains like couscous also contain protein. This one-day sample meal plan easily has over 50 grams of protein.

Could it be that you are drinking your daily calories? List any drinks you are consuming that contain calories and how frequently. What is wrong with diet drinks?

Here is an astonishing truth:

> *A large portion of the calories consumed in America now are empty calories from liquid drinks.*

A Skinny Vanilla Latte Venti made with non-fat milk and no whipped cream from Starbucks still has 160 calories! I have a patient who used to drink six or seven of these a day, even after she had her weight loss surgery. She believed she was making a good choice because they're made with non-fat milk and are called "skinny." Well, those seven "skinny" drinks still added about 1,000 calories a day to her diet! When she found out the REAL skinny on this drink, she quit her habit, and is now well on her way to weight loss success.

What about alcohol? Are you consuming empty calories with poor alcohol choices? If you don't remember the exact numbers on alcohol, please reread the sections on Basic Nutrition and Social Eating for a refresher. One margarita can pack up to 600 calories! If you are at a party and absolutely must have a drink, wine is a lower-calorie option. I love to socialize, and by no means am I a tea-totaler. I love a good party, too, but I try to keep everything in perspective and not over-indulge.

"What about all of these new-fangled, fancy-schmancy, energy drinks, Dr. Vuong?"

If you "need" them for energy, then probably either you: 1) are not getting proper nutrition, so your body is seeking that nourishment from any quickly available source; or 2) have fallen for the multi-billion-dollar marketing hype. Most of these drinks pack *a lot* of calories. They take you on a sugar high only to let you crash a couple of hours later. Remember that calories are our body's source of energy, so anything that calls itself "energy," even if it has a picture of someone running uphill on it, is going to be full of calories. There has been a lot of televised scrutiny lately of the so-called "5 hour energy shots" due to multiple deaths related to their consumption. The FDA is investigating after five deaths were linked to consumption of Monster energy drinks. Most recently, a 16 year-old girl died after consuming two 24-ounce Monsters in 24 hours, leading to caffeine toxicity ("Caffeine Questions: How Much is Too Much?", 2012.) Quite simply, I tell my patients to avoid them.

"What is the problem with diet sodas?" you ask. Plenty. Let me give you some things to think about here. One morning in my office, three new patients were sitting around the kitchen table, waiting for my dietitian to develop a 1,200-calorie meal plan with them. I came in and poured myself a small cup of coffee. I put two sugar packets in my coffee. One of the patients, whose BMI was almost 55, said to me, "Dr. Vuong, you are setting a bad example for us. You are supposed to be demonstrating healthy choices."

"What's the problem?" I asked, knowing where this conversation was heading. My current BMI is 20. I like sugar in my coffee, but I only drink one cup a day.

She said, "Why are you putting sugar packets in your coffee? That's bad for you!"

I responded with, "I know where sugar comes from—sugar cane—but I don't know where the stuff in pink, blue, or yellow packets comes from."

The truth is, it's not any one item, like sugar or butter, that causes us to be obese. It's what we do throughout the day that matters. It doesn't make sense for you to order a Big Mac, french fries, and a milkshake—these three items add up to almost 2,100 calories—and then think that you are making a good choice because you've also ordered a DIET Coke. Diet sodas are often over-consumed because people think they are harmless. But they have no nutritional value and pour a lot of chemicals into your system. I would rather enjoy a small amount of real sugar than a lot of artificial sweeteners. I believe my body knows how to process and handle sugar—I'm not sure it knows what to do with artificial sweeteners, especially not in the copious amounts that are present in the typical American diet.

The next time you are in a restaurant or at a social gathering, look around and see who is drinking diet soda. I'll bet you'll find it is mostly the overweight people. If you don't want to look like them, then don't copy their habits.

Could it be that you are not drinking enough water? How much water are you drinking a day? How much water should you be drinking a day?

Notice that each meal in the sample plan above starts with a "Big Glass of Water," not sweet tea, Gatorade, or soda.

On average the human body is about 60%-65% water—men have a slightly higher percentage than women because lean muscle (of which men typically have more) contains a much larger percentage of water (75%) than does fat (10%). Your brain is 75% water. Your blood is 83% water. Humans need to replace about 2.4 liters of water a day. If this is how we were naturally created, then shouldn't we replenish our bodies with the most natural and best option—clean water?

For those of you who say you don't like the "taste" of water, my answer is, you would love the "taste" of water if you were lost in the desert. You don't even need to be lost. Try this one experiment, if you don't believe me. Go for a walk or a hike where there are no convenience stores or drive-thru's around and bring only a bottle of water. Leave your water bottle at the starting point, do your walk, work up a sweat, and when you get back to the start, just try NOT to drink that water! You won't be able to; it will look too tempting. Do this exercise a couple of times and you'll be hooked on the "taste" of water. Why do I put "taste" in quotation marks? **Because water has no taste.** If your water has a taste, it is not pure water, and you might want to try filtering it.

How much water you should drink depends on your size and activity level, but it is usually around eight to ten, eight-ounce glasses per day. Put very simply, you should drink water whenever you are thirsty to ensure you are drinking enough of it. Start replacing one of your non-water drinks per day with water, and every week replace another until all of your drinks are water. Of course, there will be some exceptions, but drinking water should be the main way you quench your thirst.

"I heard you can drink too much water! Is this true, Dr. Vuong?"

The answer is no, not really. There is one psychological illness that drives people to drink excessive amounts of water. They will drink it from literally anywhere—directly from the tap, toilet water, doggie bowls, sewer drainage pipes, anywhere. So, unless you are drinking water from the rain gutters at your house, I think you will be ok to have that next bottle. Some people also drink too much water when they are training for a grueling athletic endeavor, such as a marathon, that makes them overly nervous about dehydration. This is extremely rare, as it requires drinking many cups of water every mile or so, which would make most people sick.

Could it be that you are not eating enough? How many times a day should you eat after gastric sleeve surgery?

We teach our patients to eat three meals a day, plus a snack if you are diabetic or are truly hungry between meals. Unlike some clinics, we teach our patients that breakfast is NOT the most important meal of the day, but we do encourage them to eat something in the morning, even if it is just a glass of water and a piece of fruit. They need to think about breakfast in a different way from what Denny's Restaurant would like. Breakfast should be something as simple as an egg or a protein drink plus a banana. I often eat freshly plucked spinach or kale leaves as I am thinning out my garden in the mornings. My daughter enjoys olives or red bell peppers for breakfast as much as she does a mango or a banana. Breakfast foods don't need to be different from other foods. In fact, I think that 15 minutes of light exercise, like stretching, jumping jacks, yoga, or mediation is probably more beneficial to our health than the typical American breakfast of cereal, donuts, or pancakes.

If you are hungry between meals, do not "tough it out" until the next mealtime. This is because after your surgery, you physically can't eat enough at one sitting to make up for that hunger craving. This will leave you very frustrated. Remember my patient who used to work all day, skip meals, and be ravenous when she got home? Don't fall into that cycle. Have the snack, and your next meal will be an appropriately sized, gastric sleeve meal. Make sense? Of course, by snack, I mean a good snack—not candy, cookies, chips, cheese crackers, or anything else that can cause your blood sugar to spike and crash. This is not a free pass to splurge. Have the rest of your breakfast banana, a handful of blueberries, or jicama sticks, for example. Remember Kizzie's Rule (the Third Rule)? Practice this rule during snacks.

What is the minimum number of calories you should consume to avoid metabolic slowdown? How can you combat a slow metabolism?

Any very low caloric diet (VLCD) requires monitoring by a physician. These are typically meal replacement diets of less than 1,000 calories per day. Let me repeat myself: These absolutely have to be monitored by a physician. An example of such a program is the Optifast 800 Meal Replacement Program, which takes patients down to 800 calories a day. The physician should perform regular, routine lab work to check your blood chemistries and your kidney and liver functions.

The medical field is pretty sure now that when caloric intake drops down to below 1,000 calories per day, human metabolism will slow down. This is a natural, evolutionary response. Think back to the caveman again. When humans had to scavenge for food that was not always readily available, our bodies became very efficient at storing energy in the form of fat to tide us through times when we might not be able to eat much for a few days. When food became scarce, our metabolism would slow down in order to conserve energy, at least until food became plentiful again. Since gastric sleeve surgery will take you down close to the 1,000-calorie threshold (I teach my patients to eat 1,100-1,200 calories a day), your body will want to go into hibernation mode. Your job is to keep this from happening. How do you do this, you ask?

With two simple steps:

- **Make sure you are getting the best nutrition you can** (Rule #2). This means eating real food, avoiding empty calories, preparing fresh meals, and buying organic foods whenever possible. This will give your body all of the micronutrients and building blocks it needs to perform its normal daily chemical reactions that keep you feeling good.

- **Exercise regularly.** This will keep your metabolism going by releasing natural hormones that control your "fight or flight" response. Ever heard of a "runner's high"? Sometimes, getting started with an exercise routine is tough, but think back about how great you felt after a workout—beyond feeling proud of accomplishing something, you probably also felt energized and alert. That's a natural response. It had very little to do with your expensive gym equipment, your personal trainer with rock hard abs, or your perfectly set iTunes playlist. It had everything to do with what a wonderful machine the human body is.

> *EXERCISE = ANY PHYSICAL ACTIVITY YOU LIKE TO DO THAT CAUSES YOU TO BREAK ONE BEAD OF SWEAT*

This could be as simple as putting on your pants, tying your shoes, or cleaning your house. If you've lost a lot of pounds and are near your goal weight, then these lower-level activities will no longer be considered exercise because they will no longer be strenuous enough to make you sweat. Switch to walking around the block, and when that becomes too easy, you will need to run. Instead of trekking through the park, you will need to go hiking. Instead of light water aerobics, you will need to swim laps. As you get thinner and fitter, you have to increase your level of physical activity continually.

Have you ever heard, "The last 20 pounds are the hardest to lose?" Wonder why this is? My guess is that people who complain about this would benefit from following the steps outlined above. The last 20 pounds are really the same as the first 20, but your body percentages are different (assuming the pounds are not comprised of excess skin, which needs to be surgically removed.) You need to keep making the healthiest choices possible all along the way.

The choices that allowed you to lose the first 50 percent of your excess weight will not be good enough to help you lose the last 50 percent. Does that make sense? You've got to kick it up a notch. If you lost 50 pounds by skipping the chips with your daily sandwich, then in order for you to lose the next 50 pounds, you will need to keep skipping the chips, but also replace the sandwich with a salad. If you lost 80 pounds by incorporating small bouts of exercise into your day, like taking the stairs, then in order for you to lose the next 80 pounds, you can't keep resting between floors. You've got to run up those stairs! You've got to try fresh veggies. You've got to try tofu, lentils, and fish. You've got to lace up the running shoes and go pound some pavement! Don't worry, you don't have to do all of these things at once, but just keep doing more the leaner and healthier you become.

Are you consuming empty calories (calories without any nutritious value)? Any at all? Write down everything you have eaten since breakfast yesterday morning and evaluate your choices.

If you are not losing weight, and especially if you are GAINING weight, then you are consuming too many extra calories—pure and simple.

If you want longterm weight-loss success, then you really must keep a food diary. There are no excuses when you keep a food diary—the evidence is right there in front of you. Our minds subconsciously try to ameliorate our feelings to avoid hurting us psychologically, and sometimes this can undermine our weight-loss efforts. Remember that time you were going to eat just one Girl Scout cookie, and before you knew it, the whole box was gone, and you didn't even realize it? Why was that? How did that happen? If you know that you will be accountable for every cookie, it's not as easy to keep eating. When you know that you will have to count up all the empty slots in that cookie box and then calculate how many calories the missing cookies contain and write it in your food diary, you'll find yourself able to stop after one or two, or maybe you won't even open the box at all.

People who have excellent and lasting weight loss are often the ones who keep food diaries. They are dedicated to writing down not only the calories they consume, but also the activities they do, AND all of the emotions they were feeling at the time of eating or exercising. Technology makes this easy to do. There are lots of websites with resources and references to help you log everything. There are even mobile apps that allow you to log your food intake on the spot! But some people still enjoy a plain paper notebook. One time, I saw a television news story about a woman who had lost 150 pounds without surgery. Her technique was simply to pack all of her food for the day into a small box. She could not eat anything unless it came out of that box, except for water. While this sounds extreme, it was very effective. But when I stop and think about it, that "food box" was basically the equivalent of her food diary, just manifested into a practical form that worked for her. Instead of writing down what she ate after the fact, she preemptively logged her intake before she ate by packing her entire day's worth of food into a small box.

Keeping a food journal is like anything else—it's a little difficult to get started, but once you get going, it just becomes second nature. Saying goodbye to those pounds forever is worth that extra bit of effort.

What's So Wrong With ____?

"What's So Wrong With _____?" (Quiz)

What's so wrong with BREAD?

What's so wrong with MILK?

What's so wrong with SKINLESS, BONELESS CHICKEN BREAST?

What's so wrong with WHITE RICE?

What's so wrong with FROZEN MEALS LIKE LEAN CUISINE® OR HEALTHY CHOICE®?

What's so wrong with the $1 MENU?

"What's So Wrong With _____?" (Answers)

What's so wrong with BREAD?

Once I saw a speaker at a conference pass around a McDonald's Happy Meal. It looked a little stale, but was definitely recognizable as a Happy Meal. The hamburger bun seemed bouncy, the meat gray, and the french fries had a slight smell of grease. He then asked us how old we thought that Happy Meal was. Most people in the audience guessed one week or one month. Someone had the audacity to guess six months. Imagine our surprise when he passed around the original receipt that was dated EIGHT YEARS earlier! Why won't it decay? McDonald's food is so bad that not even mold will eat it.

Just as the Happy Meal shares few properties with real food, the modern version of bread bears very little resemblance to the breads that nourished our forefathers. Historically, bread was baked daily. This is because freshly baked bread will grow stale in one to two days. After that, it is too hard to eat by itself. At this point, the bread is often used as a serving vessel for soup or is used for something else, like croutons or breadcrumbs. Have you ever wondered how it is possible for store-bought, modern bread to have a shelf life of up to six weeks? The processing of the flour removes all of the nutrition, and added preservatives give it shelf life. One of the main preservatives used is salt, so

> *Bread is the #1 source of sodium in the American diet.*

—not because of the percentage of salt in it, but due to the fact that we eat so much bread! Have you ever wondered why the package says, "enriched white bread"? If bread nourished our forefathers during times of war and got many Americans through the Great Depression, then why does today's bread have to be enriched? It is because all of the nutrition has been removed to give it shelf life.

The other problem with bread is that it is ubiquitous in our society. It's usually served with each meal—and in ridiculous proportions, too. No one should be eating a 12 inch sandwich on a regular basis or consuming a double-meat hamburger or medium pizza on their own. If you want to be healthier, you should try to avoid bread most days, in all of its forms. Here is a short list of some food items that you probably never thought of as BREAD, but that all function the same way nutritionally:

Breakfast—pancakes, waffles, toast, cereals, croissants, muffins, bagels, breakfast bars, danishes, and pastries
Lunch—sandwich bread, hamburger buns, hot dog buns, giant pretzels, pizza crust, flour tortillas, pasta
Snack—plain crackers, chips, cookies, peanut crackers, etc...
Dinner—dinner rolls, bread sticks, side of white bread, instant pasta, cakes, pie crusts

BREAD IS NOT YOUR FRIEND.

What's so wrong with MILK?

The American dairy industry and most Americans would disagree with me, but I think no one in America should be drinking milk on a daily basis. The only person in America who should be drinking cow's milk on a daily basis is a baby cow, and here's why:

Milk is relatively high in fat content. The dairy industry has done such a great job that we think we all need to have milk moustaches! "Don't I need it for calcium, Dr. Vuong?" you ask. There are better and less fatty options for calcium, like broccoli. I think the health cost of milk is too high a price to pay for the nutrition you're getting. In terms of your health, it is a very expensive milk moustache.

Dairy cows are given a tremendous amount of hormones in order to continuously produce milk. They are often hooked up to the pumps all day long. This is unnatural. And the hormones are making their way into our food supply. Studies suggest this is possibly one reason why the age of menarche (a girl's first menstrual cycle) is dropping (Wiley, 2011.) It's not unusual now to hear about elementary school children starting menstruation or about a fifth grade girl having a baby! Imagine if you are the parent of that girl. Isn't forgoing milk a small price for giving children back the chance to experience childhood?

Dairy cows are injected with antibiotics. Sores develop on their teets from being kept on the suction pumps for so long. These sores get infected, and the pus from those infections ends up in the milk supply. Dairy farmers are allowed to have a certain level of measurable pus in the milk, and they give the dairy cows antibiotics to keep them alive and to keep the infections from inhibiting their milk supply (Pilzer, 82-85.) The infected pus in the milk leads to a major immune response in our bodies. We have a serious problem with milk allergies now in America. And the consumption of the antibiotics that pass into the milk supply (and into meat supplies as well) reduces the effectiveness of antibiotics we need to take for our own infections. When you are really sick, you want your antibiotics to work, which they won't do effectively if we've already bred bacteria with immunity to them.

What's so wrong with SKINLESS, BONELESS CHICKEN BREAST?

Skinless, boneless chicken breast is one of America's most favorite kitchen staples, so what I say next will surprise many professional dieters: **I am not a big fan of skinless, boneless, chicken breast.** Here's why:

Skinless, boneless chicken breast lacks flavor. I guess that's why many people like to use it as an ingredient—it is widely tolerated by most palettes. But I like to taste my food. Since the skinless, boneless breast is a bland starting point for a dish, you have to add sauces for flavor. How often have you said, "I don't know what else to do with this chicken breast." Or your family has said, "Aw, chicken breast again?" Change it up—try something with more innate flavor, like duck, Cornish hen, quail, or even pheasant.

Skinless, boneless, chicken breast tends to dry out, especially if it is reheated. This could make it hard for you as a patient to ingest past your sleeve. It also makes it hard to repurpose or reuse later. I suggest to my patients that they do not bring home their chicken dinner leftovers for themselves (a doggy bag for the doggy is great, though!)

The main reason I don't like skinless, boneless chicken breast is because it is more processed than a whole chicken, and I teach my patients to avoid processed foods as much as possible. From least to most processed chicken, the progression is:

Whole chicken➔Whole cut up chicken➔Separated chicken sections (quarters, halves)➔Separated chicken pieces (all thighs or all breasts)➔Bone-in, skin-on breasts➔ Boneless, skinless chicken breasts➔chicken tenders

Each time you move down the arrow, the meat you are buying gets separated, processed, and handled more and more. Because of the additional labor needed for each step, you end up paying an inordinately high price for the chicken tenders, which are essentially nothing more than the underside of the breast meat. A whole chicken costs roughly $5, but six little tender strips often cost $7 or $8. There is no reason why you can't buy a whole chicken and separate it yourself. It would take under two minutes and save you a lot of money. I prefer to roast the whole chicken first (it has good flavor and is juicy), then use any leftovers for other meals. In a pinch, I will buy a whole rotisserie chicken that has already been cooked. How easy is that? And you can buy them for about $6 each!

What's so wrong with WHITE RICE?

Some people may think that I have a natural bias for white rice because I am Asian. They might be correct, but I just don't believe that white rice is the enemy that all the dieting tips suggest, and I have over a billion data points to prove it. There are more than one billion Asians across the world who eat white rice daily, sometimes three times a day, and are much healthier than most Westerners. They also eat white rice in the form of rice noodles, rice cakes, rice soups, and even rice desserts. While it's true that brown rice has more nutrients than white, I do not believe that simply changing the color of your rice is going to have any significant impact on your health.

What Asians don't do is cover rice with heavy sauces like gravy, butter, or cream. White rice is plentiful in the typically economically poorer Asian regions, while meat is scarce. Authentic Asian cuisine includes a main entrée that is usually intense in flavor, but it is proportionately small compared to the amount of rice that accompanies it. Westerners often describe these entrées as pungent. Think of the fish sauce, soy sauce, or shrimp paste that flavors the meat dish. The white rice helps to spread the meal over a large group of people. Often, one chicken can feed a family of five for a few days. Overall, they are consuming fewer calories, even though they eat a lot of rice.

A culture and its people make the most of the readily available resources. For example, most days, Asians will eat white rice. During holidays or on special occasions, they will make special, stir-fried rice. On the other hand, when Americans go to Chinese restaurants, most will order stir-fried rice with their entrée (which is usually intended to be family style, but is rarely eaten as such) because it is readily available on the menu. One serving of white rice has about 150 calories, but a serving of stir-fried rice can have 600 calories! I once saw an obese couple order a platter of fried rice each in addition to their "healthy Chinese entrée". Each fried rice platter probably had at least eight servings! Eating such a platter is akin to having eight sodas at one meal instead of just on occasion.

What's so wrong with FROZEN MEALS LIKE LEAN CUISINE® OR HEALTHY CHOICE®?

Many dieters find these frozen "meals" convenient and believe that they are literally making a healthy choice if they have them for lunch. A technique touted by many diet programs is to substitute your typical fast food or cafeteria lunch for one of these "healthier" frozen meals. And maybe for the first week or two, the dieter does find it convenient, likes the selections, and maybe even loses a few pounds. But inevitably, the selections will get stale, the routine will be interrupted by meetings and outings, and the weight loss will stop. Once she quits using the frozen entrees, she finds that the weight comes back on, and often more than she lost.

The majority of these dieting meals work because they limit portion size. Rarely are they actually healthier for you. Once you open the package, the meal never looks as large or pretty as the picture on the package, does it? You take the meal out of the package, hoping that heating it up will make it look more like the tempting picture, then take it out of the microwave, and to your surprise, all you see is an amorphous glop of food product covered in a thick sauce. The vegetables taste bland and boiled. The chicken is rubbery. The "dessert" usually tastes sweet, but not decadent.

In order to combat this perceived paucity, Lean Cuisine now has a line of larger meals that have a 30 percent larger portion size. Again, the companies are successfully catering to consumer wants, but not to their health. In order to freeze these meals and have them reheat to a palatable level, they are often loaded with preservatives, like salt. There are "flavor enhancers," "artificial colorings," and "food stabilizers". Do any of those sound healthy?

To keep these "meals" profitable, companies have to source the most cost-effective ingredients. In other words, they find the cheapest ingredients they can. In order to scale a business, the company has to be able to reduce the unit price of each product to a certain amount; otherwise, they cannot make any money.

In the end, it will be cheaper, easier, tastier, and healthier if you just pack a big salad with a wide selection of fruits and vegetables and some lean protein. You will feel great if you choose this simple option for lunch every day and finally get off the frozen entrée train ride.

What's so wrong with the $1 MENU?

Many Americans think that they are getting a great deal at the drive-thru. After all, the "$1 Value Menu" or "Value Deal" must be a great deal, right? Well, not so fast. You really should reconsider this "value" proposition the next time you are tempted to take your children, the softball team, or the scout troop there. Here's why:

Poor Quality of "Food" — How can anyone or any company possibly make a hamburger for $1? Think about it. It's impossible to do so...unless you use the cheapest grade of meat and the lowest quality of bread, and you minimize the toppings. Have you ever looked at the color and texture of the meat patty on a $1 hamburger? When you pull the patty apart, is it juicy and delicate or is it gray and sinewy? Gray and sinewy means it was made from the cheapest scraps of meat, full of gristle and connective tissue. The airiness of the bun means it was made from the most highly processed white flour. The fact that it only has two pickles (if any at all) means that the company was trying to put a non-perishable item on your burger to add a little burst of flavor. You couldn't use lettuce — it would wilt, look bad, and not add much flavor.

"But Dr. Vuong, where else can I get full so cheaply?" This is a misleading type of thinking that contributes to the obesity problem. First, even though it's called the "$1 Menu," seldom do you leave paying just $1. The food companies know this, and they don't become multi-million (or –billion) dollar corporations from their $1 menus. It's rare these days to go through the drive-thru and pay less than $7-8/person. Second, the nutritional value of the meal is often so low that your body starts running out of energy later on in the day. Ever wonder why, after a big, fast food meal, you are hungry again at 3:00 or 4:00 in the afternoon? Now you've got to go pay for a snack. Add that all up, and hopefully you'll see how little value you actually got. That's even before considering the cost to your health!

But here is the worst thing about ordering from the $1 Menu. If you regularly order from this selection, then **you are subconsciously telling yourself that you are worth only $1.** Get it? You might not realize it, but you are. Subconsciously, this choice represents a "Poor Mentality" instead of an "Abundance Mentality." It is an "I'm not worth it" mindset, as opposed to a "You cannot put a price on my health" mentality. It says, "I value myself at $1" and not "I deserve only the best." These are two very different ways of thinking, and over time, one will lead to obesity and feelings of inadequacy, while the other will lead to success and fulfillment.

If you take your children and tell them to order from the $1 Menu, then you let them know that you think they are worth only $1. Now, I know no parent does this on purpose, but that is still the message you are sending. This will dramatically affect their lives. They will subconsciously think, "I'm only worth $1, so it's ok if I let other kids pick on me." "We've never had much, so I don't feel right taking this opportunity." "It (the soccer uniform, musical instrument, college, studying abroad) costs too much." "I can't do it; let me go the cheap and easy route." "I don't matter much—I'm only worth $1." This is a Poor Mentality that will do great damage to their lives.

So choose yourself and your family over the "Value" Menu.

Healthy Shopping Skills

Healthy Shopping Skills (Quiz)

Name three "impulse" items located in the store that you struggle with.

Identify one tactic to reduce "temptation" or "impulse" shopping.

Give an example of why buying in bulk can work against your weight management goals.

List three ways to save money and shop in a healthier way at the grocery store.

Why are terms such as "sugar-free," "sugarless," "low fat," and "all-natural" misleading?

When reading labels, what should you focus on?

What would be a healthier choice for the food selections listed below?

Whole milk—

Butter—

Cheese—

White rice—

White bread—

Lunch meat—

List one unhealthy shopping habit that you have and explain how you will change it.

Will you commit to this change TODAY?

What is the First Rule of WLS Eating?

Healthy Shopping Skills (Answers)

Name three "impulse" items located in the store that you struggle with.

Has this ever happened to you? You head out on a quick trip to the grocery store for some toilet paper, milk, or whatever little item you need. You dash through the store to get the item you need so you can make it back home in time for *The Voice*, but wait a minute! The bag of chips, your favorite cookies, or the Diet Coke® is on sale, or if you buy one, you'll get the second one free. You've got to buy it, right? It's just too good of a deal! And why is that sale item always at the end of the aisle, so that in your rush to turn the corner, you always happen to run into it? That store manager should really do a better job of placing his sale items in a proper place so that shoppers who are in a hurry, like you, aren't slowed down when you run into them. You would stop to give him this suggestion, if you weren't already so late. When you're walking to your car, instead of just a gallon of milk, you notice you have a whole bag of stuff!

Impulse buying can be significant, like this, or the simple act of buying a candy bar while you're waiting in line, or grabbing a Starbucks (often "conveniently" located inside the grocery store) to drink while you shop.

It is really imperative that you learn all of the stocking tricks that grocery stores use to get you to buy more. These are proven methods—developed over the years by marketing research firms—that they employ on you! Ever wonder why the cheap, individually wrapped, easy-to-pick-up gum, candy, batteries, etc., are at the checkout line? Ever notice that the sugary cereals are at your kids' eye level, and all of the healthy stuff is up high, down low, or even in an entirely different section of the store? Did you know that producers pay more money to have grocery chains stock their items in these prime locations? It is no coincidence that you enter a store only wanting to buy some milk and leave with a bag full of treats.

Identify one tactic to reduce "temptation" or "impulse" shopping.

You will find endless lists available on the Net and Web forums on this topic. It seems like every New Year's, there's a story on this topic, adapted to the current atmosphere. After the economic downturn, it seemed like I saw several articles on "How to shop on a budget without ruining your diet," or something to that effect. The tips are usually a rehash of the same old stuff. But in case you've never seen one, here are some tips to help you get started:

- Don't shop when you're hungry.
- Make a list so know what you need and buy *only* what you need.
- Walk the perimeter of the store where the fresh produce, meats, and fish are.
- Look up and down (tempting items that you don't need are usually placed at eye level and the ends of aisles).
- Avoid interior aisles all together.
- Make shopping a learning experience with your young kids, nieces and nephews, or the neighbors. This is what I do with my child.
  - o You can point out the names of the fresh produce, and discuss their origins. That's a good way to practice geography since most stores sell produce that comes from all over the world.
  - o Practice math by showing them how to weigh the items and figure out the cost.
  - o Teach them proper serving sizes in order to plan meals.
  - o Teach them about making a purchase. My daughter, Kizzie, earns her own money doing chores. I allow her to make purchases with her money at the grocery store as she sees fit. Yes, she may choose jelly beans, but buying jelly beans once in a while becomes a big occasion and not something that automatically happens. I also allow her to hand the money to the cashier and to receive the change. She is required to say, "Thank you." Most people in line smile when they see my little girl painstakingly count out all of her dimes and nickels, trying to save as many of her quarters as possible.

Give an example of why buying in bulk can work against your weight management goals.

I have many friends who swear by the savings found in big warehouse stores like Sam's Club or Costco, but unless you own a small business, I don't really understand the benefits of shopping at one of these stores. Ask yourself whether you really need to have all of the extra food lying around. If it is in your home, it will be readily available to eat when you're just a little tired or stressed, and most of the bulk items are "snack foods", not ingredients that can be used to cook healthy meals. What I have found when perusing these stores is that most of the items have a shelf life, which means they are processed and, hence, not what I consider to be real food. While some have meats and seafood, most of the meat is not good quality and most of the seafood is frozen. Much of the fruit or produce is not any cheaper than that in the regular stores. Next time you are there, just take a peak at what is in other peoples' carts. Ask yourself, "Is this REAL food that I am providing for my family?"

As I've mentioned before, Hurricane Ike came through Galveston in September 2008 and devastated lots of homes. My neighborhood was under seven feet of water in most places, including inside my home. We were without power for almost one month. Many people returned to their homes and discovered tons of rotten and spoiled foods in their freezers and refrigerators. The stench was unbearable the first few days after the hurricane. Residents had to throw out multiple freezers full of bad food, spoiled hunting meat, and rotten fish from multiple fishing trips. As I drove around, I asked myself, why did these people need so much food? Especially frozen food? Did they know something that I did not? Were they hoarding food for a reason? Perhaps the last problem we have in this country is a shortage of available food.

As I write, Hurricane Sandy has recently devastated the northeastern seaboard, and the scene has been reminiscent of what I went through with Hurricane Ike, except on an even larger scale. Those long lines of people waiting to get ice and water—not food—reappeared. People were complaining about the lack of fresh drinking water—not soda, Gatorade, or food, but just water. When fresh water is scarce, this simplest of resources can no longer be taken for granted.

There is also another problem with having large quantities of food lying around. Studies have shown that we will eat more if a larger portion size is placed in front of us (CDC, Division of Nutrition and Physical Activity, 2006.) So if you buy a big jug or container of something, you will most likely consume it all AND in the same amount of time as you would a smaller jug or container of the same item. For example, if you buy a jumbo container of pretzels, you will most likely eat them in the same amount of time that it would have taken to eat a small bag. In other words, if you are buying a big supply of food, thinking it will last longer or that it will somehow save you time by decreasing your trips to the store, you're fooling yourself. You will probably end up eating more of almost anything processed—chips, cookies, soda, etc. But this probably isn't the case for fresh fruit and vegetables—they will probably spoil. Why would your kids choose to eat fresh fruit when there is a huge bag of cookies right next to it?

So, the next time you go shopping, consider this: Is the money you're saving (and even that point is debatable) really worth the harm you are doing to your body or to your family? At best, I think it is a shift of money—a possible "savings" at the grocery store that you end up paying out at the doctor's office, pharmacy, or hospital.

List three ways to save money and shop in a healthier way at the grocery store.

Everyone thinks I'm crazy, but I shop for one meal at a time. If I am feeling particularly adventurous that day, I might shop for two meals, like dinner that night and brunch the next day. Even with my hectic schedule, I still find time to cook four or five dinners every week for my family. People ask me how I find time. I respond, "How do you NOT have time?" I just make it a priority. It is important to me to provide my family with fresh, healthy meals as frequently as possible. This is a way that I show them my love. I don't mean cooking them deep-fried, greasy foods in huge proportions that bust open their belts. That's not love, in my opinion; that is killing them slowly with food. I don't have snacks lying around, either—if I shop every day, I don't need "handy (pre-packaged) snacks", because I always have fresh food available. But if you are going to be a frequent flyer at the grocery store, there are some things you need to know.

162

Avoid marketing gimmicks, like "New and Improved," "Even Cheesier," "30% more FREE," "Buy 2, Get 1 Free" (unless there are bargains on non-perishable items, like toilet paper, of course.) There will always be something on sale or something improved, and it is more economical overall to stick to what you need.

Buy just what you need for your meals. If you are buying fresh, then you should only be shopping around the perimeter of the store. A lot of patients are surprised by how much money they save when they pass on the frozen meals, the extra snacks, the bottled drinks, and the unnecessary impulse buys.

Make your cashier work, because it means you are buying fresh. Every produce item has been given a universal four-digit code that identifies it. The code is often located on a small sticker that is on the piece of produce. Cashiers must learn these codes in order to register the sale. If the sticker falls off and they do not know the code by memory, then they usually have to look it up on a laminated picture sheet or list. Most cashiers will have memorized the common items, like bananas, but not the less frequently purchased items, like taro root. I always make it a goal to purchase items that make my cashier have to work a little extra by entering in the code, rather than just mindlessly scanning packaged products, like frozen dinners. Even better if they learn the name of a mysterious vegetable in the process. Besides, they always get a little chuckle, when, as they are searching for the number, I tell them the code for ginger root is 4612.

Buy organic foods. I know what you are thinking, because I thought the same thing initially. Why should I pay $2.99 a pound for organic broccoli (or apples, or any other item) when regular broccoli is only $1.99 a pound? Organic foods can be two, three, or four times as expensive as the conventional variety. Today I bought organic bone-in chicken breast for $8.99 per pound when the regular chicken breast next to it was only $4.99. But the difference in nutritional value for certain vitamins and minerals can be many times greater in organic foods, easily justifying their higher price (Oliveira, 2013.) And that doesn't even take into account all the chemicals you avoid by eating organic foods. So, I just decided that I am worth that extra dollar or two for my organic broccoli, especially since it seems like the prices for organic foods are coming down a little every year (or maybe the conventional prices are just rising—but either way, the disparity between the prices is shrinking). More importantly, I decided that my family is worth it. If you forgo that package of cookies, you'll be able to buy organic and still save money.

Avoid items with a shelf life. These foods are highly processed and injected or coated with preservatives and chemicals that you just don't need. They have to be in order to even have a "shelf life." This is done so that mold won't begin to break them down. If mold won't eat them, then why should you?

Why are terms such as "sugar-free," "sugarless," "low fat," and "all-natural" misleading?

These labels are mostly marketing ploys without any real meaning behind them. Most of the time, these labels don't address the actual nutritional value of food. Also, if these "foods" have packages on which manufacturers can place labels, then they are probably processed and, therefore, are not real foods that you should be eating.

> *A piece of fruit is far more natural than anything in a box claiming to be all-natural.*

On meat and poultry packages, "all-natural," "hormone-free," and other such labels have various meanings, but none of them carry as much weight as "Organic". A chicken that is raised in a small and filthy coop, injected with antibiotics, and fed "food" that no chicken has business eating can be labeled "all-natural." What is "natural" after all? There is no regulation on what counts as "natural", and anyone can apply that and other similar terms to their products. However, the label "USDA-Certified Organic" means that the chicken was raised in a clean environment, fed USDA-Certified Organic feed, not injected with antibiotics, treated humanely, and raised according to a number of other standards, including fair labor laws. No sewage sludge can be used as a fertilizer for organic produce, no food can be irradiated or bioengineered, and growing methods have to be environmentally sustainable or "green". Furthermore, government officials have checked the facility on a regular basis to ensure that it meets these criteria. There are very few cases of fraudulent organic labeling, because not only does the government monitor this label, but other organic farmers monitor it. They want consumers to feel secure that their products are better than the non-organic versions so that they can charge more for them. These higher prices cover the farmers' higher costs in raising their animals in these more humane ways. Consumer advocacy groups also verify that the organic labeling is justified. There is a lot of internal regulation taking place that makes that organic seal significant. "Organic", therefore, is the only food claim I would hang my hat on, although "Local" or "Locally Grown" have also become popular buzz words lately.

On most weekends and in most cities and many small towns across the United States, you can find a local farmer's market or cooperative now. The Locally Grown movement has really caught on. Rice University has a farmer's market every Tuesday in the parking lot of the football stadium, right in the middle of Houston! Many farmers are placing fruit and vegetable stands and market areas along highways. Restaurants are partnering with area farmers to get the freshest in-season produce possible, and many chefs are changing their menus regularly to take advantage of regionally available products. This is often called "farm-to-table dining." I think it is great that American society is becoming more aware of the global impact of our eating, farming, and commerce habits.

When reading labels, what should you focus on?

This is somewhat of a trick question. If the food has a nutrition label, then you probably shouldn't eat it, or at least not eat it on a regular basis. Remember, it's the everyday things we do that matter. So, if every evening, you settle down for a bedtime snack, the fact that you are eating it every night before bed trumps whatever its nutritional label claims. If you eat a low-fat yogurt with "real fruit" at the bottom and lots of calcium every night, you are also eating about 100 extra calories and a lot of sugars or chemicals. You'd be better off forgoing that yogurt. Do you see my point? **If you eat real food regularly and labeled food sparingly, you will reach your weight loss and health goals.**

If you insist on reading food labels, then here is the information you should focus on:

- Look at the number of calories, but also note the serving size—a single cookie could in fact be labeled as two servings, so you would need to double the calorie and fat quantities if you expect to eat the whole cookie. One serving of Ramen noodles is actually only half of the package, not the entire little package! So if you eat the entire package (which is what most people do), then you would consume 380 calories and 70 percent of your daily allowance for salt.

- Be careful of the salt and fat content.
- The more recognizable terms, the better.
- The shorter the list, the better.
- And remember the First Rule? Note the protein content.

What would be a healthier choice for the food selections listed below?

Whole milk—Soy milk is a much better choice. Remember this the next morning you are thirsty: an eight-ounce glass of whole milk has the equivalent of a pat of butter in it. Soy milk is a great source of protein with very little fat and no hormones. Calcium is added to soy milk to give it the same level that is found in milk.

Butter—Olive oil is better, but butter is still better than margarine. I don't know what margarine is made of, so definitely avoid it. Lard is also worse than butter. I often cook with a little pat of butter mixed in olive oil. I use the olive oil for its high burning temperature and butter for its flavor. One little pat of butter is not the enemy, especially when it means my family will enjoy the green beans I'm sauteeing. The enemy is the multiple sticks of butter that go into making that Italian cream cake!

Cheese—Buy REAL cheese, the stuff from the deli that costs $10 for an eight-ounce block. Use it to augment your meal (like a serving of fruit and cheese as an appetizer), not as the main ingredient in a dish like lasagna, cheese enchiladas, or mac and cheese. Real cheese should have about seven grams of protein per ounce. Do not use anything labeled "processed cheese food". This is a product made mostly from hydrogenated oils. In Europe, people have to go to school in order to become a cheese-maker. After school, they take an apprenticeship with an established cheese-maker to practice the art of making delicate cheeses. They have to learn the slight nuances of each cheese. For example, most cheeses have to be turned by hand daily. And making a cheese could take a year or more depending on how they are aged. On the other hand, most American cheeses are made in big factories, using pasteurized milk, so that the cheese can be ready to sell in six weeks or less.

This difference in attention to detail and craftsmanship dramatically affects the flavor of the cheese. Real cheese is far more flavorful, and among French cheeses alone, there are more varieties than there are days in a year!

White rice—Plain white rice is better than rice that comes with an added "flavoring" packet, but brown rice is nutritionally better than white. Couscous, quinoa, and simple polenta are even better choices because they contain more nutrients and fiber. But I think white rice has gotten a bad rap in the diet community. As an Asian immigrant to this country, I have mixed feelings when I hear people say that white rice is unhealthy. This is because I have over one billion brothers and sisters across the globe who are thin and healthy, and they eat white rice two or three times a day. But how we Asians eat and prepare our rice is very different from how Americans do it. I discuss this in this the section titled, "What's So Wrong With____?"

White bread—no bread is best, but wheat bread or multi-grain bread is better than white. Be careful, though, as some "wheat" breads are merely white breads with a "drop" of wheat content and some brown food coloring. Choose breads with a fiber content of at least three grams per slice. But no matter what type of bread you choose, if you as an adult are eating a sandwich made with two slices of bread everyday for lunch, you will probably be overweight in a few years. This is especially true if most of your sandwiches come from storefronts or fast food restaurants—the serving sizes are just way too big. No one other than a professional athlete should be eating a 12-inch sandwich on a regular basis!

Lunch meat—Lunch meats are filled with preservatives and flavorings, so buy real cooked meats, like roasted chicken. Have you ever stopped and wondered exactly what is in bologna that gives it that particular special shade of lavender pink and gummy texture? It is a highly processed product. What does that even mean, you ask? Well, this means that the typical bologna we loved as kids comes from the conveyor belt after-thoughts of the meat industry—things like organs, trimmings, end pieces, and so on. They are all ground together, doused with some chemicals and colorings, and formed and cut into round slices. If you watched bologna being made, you'd probably never eat it again.

List one unhealthy shopping habit that you have and explain how you will change it.

This is a personal answer, but we all could do better. Take me as an example. For special occasions and parties, I used to buy a chocolate mousse pie from the bakery. I liked it so much that one weekday, I bought it to have for dessert after dinner. My family and I ate pieces of it for a couple of days and were happy. I then started trying the different pies and cakes the bakery had to offer, and before I knew it, I bought dessert on almost every shopping trip. It wasn't until Melissa started complaining about her figure that I made the connection—and I do this for a living folks! Now we save the pies for very special occasions and eat fresh fruit after dinner every night.

You probably know what you are doing wrong in the shopping department. Are you buying too many prepackaged foods, sweets, sodas, chips, artificially-flavored foods, or impulse treats in too great of a quantity? Are you not buying enough fresh fruits and vegetables, real meats, or other real foods that spoil?

Here is an easy tip: **Add one good item to your cart now BEFORE you start taking away a bad item.** Do this regularly and before you know it, your cart will be full of MOSTLY good items. Now just be sure to **eat those good items** once you get home!

Will you commit to this change TODAY?

Why wait any longer? Make changes that matter now. Quit fretting about it. Quit worrying about what your family will think or what your kids will say. Quit worrying about what your friends will do or your coworkers will mention. None of it matters. Take action today. Do something for yourself.

What is the First Rule of WLS Eating?

"Protein First" applies not just to how you eat, but also to how you shop. That means go pick up your protein first, be it a meat or nonanimal source, then your fruits and veggies (the Second and Third Rules), then your essential non-perishables, and then if you have any money left, you can maybe get a non-essential item. If you are preparing fresh meals with a focus on good protein, then it only makes sense that you follow this shopping order. This is how I shop. I always shop with a meal in mind, plus a back-up plan. I go to the meat and fish department first to look for the lamb chops or whole tilapia, and if they aren't carrying what I need, then I adjust my meal plan. Then I plan my side dishes. Then I pick up the paper towels, trash bags, or soap, or whatever household goods I need, pay for my items, and leave the store. Shopping this way does not take long, and I can always use the express lane. You will either have to pay for fresh groceries or medical bills and medicines. The choice is yours.

I like to think of my fresh groceries as my first line of preventive medicine!

Holiday Eating Tips

Happy holidays—whether it's the 4th of July, Thanksgiving, a family reunion, or your yearly cruise! Congratulations for wanting to maintain healthy eating strategies during this time. Below are some good rules for anyone who wants to maintain their weight during the food-filled holidays. After these, I add some extra tips specifically for gastric sleeve patients.

Don't Start a Diet

Dieting during the holidays or while on a vacation almost never works. It will not only frustrate you, and also detract from the key aspect of the holidays—to celebrate family bonds, enjoy yourself and the company of others, and make new and lasting memories. TV shows that have a segment on "How to make your Thanksgiving healthier" or "How to avoid ruining your diet during the holidays" promote backwards thinking. I've waited all year for my sweet potato pie, and now the "diet expert" is going to mess it up by substituting low-fat yogurt instead of cream? I don't think so. We should feel free to celebrate holidays as we choose. In terms of weight loss, it's the rest of the year that matters, not these special times. Instead, **make it a goal to maintain your weight.** This will allow you to enjoy holidays or vacation while remaining mindful of your health. If you still lose weight, like several of my gastric sleeve patients have done, then that's a bonus, but it doesn't need to be your primary goal.

Eat a Light Snack Before You Go

If you are going to a party, **eat ahead of time**. Saving "room" for all the great food is nothing but a recipe for disaster. If you arrive at a party hungry, chances are, you will choose calorie-dense foods, which are often prevalent at celebrations. This is a natural, biological response. Instead, try eating enough healthy food beforehand so that you're satisfied before you arrive. You'll have much more self-control around those tempting party treats, and you will have given your body the nutrients it needs (no, your body does not need anything found in a slice of pie).

Give Up the "I've Already Blown It" Mentality

Have you ever thought, "I've already ruined my diet today (or this week or this month), so it doesn't matter what I eat now!"? There are times when we all make poor food choices, but that doesn't mean you have to throw in the towel! This is one of the few times in life that we behave this way. University of Pennsylvania psychologist Judith S. Beck suggests: Pretend you get pulled over for running a red light, and the police officer gives you a ticket. At this point, you wouldn't say, "Well I've blown it now. I might as well just run all of the other red lights today!" If you stumble down the first couple of steps on a flight of stairs, you wouldn't think, "Well, I've blown it now!" and throw yourself down the rest of the staircase! So why do we do this with our food choices? I think it's because **the consequences of our bad food choices aren't immediately apparent**, unlike the lecture and ticket from the police officer for running red lights or the bruises and broken bones from falling down stairs. If you eat a pound of cookies, you won't immediately gain a pound. If you skip your run around the park, you won't get dimples on your thighs that night. No, health consequences are slow and insidious. We often think of dieting as a Good-Bad option, but living a healthy lifestyle is much more than that and requires an understanding of your role in this world. The personal benefits of healthy choices are small and incremental, not sudden and immediate. You need to think of making healthy choices as your regular daily routine as opposed to something out of the norm. And never, ever feel that if one day you eat a plate of pasta with a diet soda and then go through a big chocolate bar while lying on the couch that you have failed! Doing it once is not an excuse to do it again. Everybody falls off the wagon sometimes. The important question is, "What am I going to do from this point forward?"

Step back from the situation, reassess, acknowledge the choice you made, and then move forward with a renewed commitment to do better. It's never too late to stop, and it's nothing to be ashamed about. The only way to **turn your healthy choices into good habit** is by continuing to make them, despite the changing scenario. You need to continue to consciously choose to make them regardless of the "little challenges" we all face on a daily basis. Keep in mind that weight is based on calories consumed and calories expended, so every decision you make matters. Everyone overeats sometimes, but your goal is to contain the damage already done, not give up or decide that the whole week is blown and plan to get back on track on Monday. Keeping a food diary will keep you accountable for all those calories that might seem as though they don't count because you eat them after you've already splurged. But stopping a splurge before you order a second margarita is far better than going ahead with a second, third, and fourth!

Plan Ahead

Think about what you are going to eat when you get to a party or family gathering. Even go so far as to write down what you will eat. This will empower you to take control of the situation, and **empowerment is the key to success in all things**, not just weight loss. It will help you to remain conscious of your choices and to avoid slipping into mindless eating patterns.

Life is too short to live it mindlessly!

You'll feel even more accountable if you go back to your list and write down what you actually did eat and compare your choices with your plan. For many patients, knowing what to eat becomes routine for them, and they don't need to actively plan as much. For some patients, it is something they continue to do.

Know Who the "Saboteurs" Are

Every family has someone who tries, deliberately or not, to sabotage others' weight loss efforts. Have a response ready for these people who try to tempt you with sweets and treats. The truth that you are trying to make healthier choices usually works well. But sometimes, the saboteur will still push that chicken-fried steak in front of you anyway. Here are a few lines that my patients have told me are really hard for any saboteur not to heed:

- "I have blood work for my (physical, annual, etc.) on Monday, and my doctor told me that (tempting item) could ruin the results."
- "I have a toothache right now."
- "I was told that food type would interfere with some medication I am taking."
- "My husband and I have a tradition of sharing dessert alone with each other every holiday, so I am saving up for that later tonight, but thanks anyway!"

Then hopefully, the saboteur will try to help your efforts, not hinder them. Besides, once you give some compelling reason why you can't have that treat, you probably won't feel comfortable changing your mind later and having to explain yourself!

Enlist an Army of More Than One

Going at it by yourself can be lonely, so **get the support of your friends and family**. Talk openly about the healthy changes you're making and try to encourage them to do the same. I always encourage my patients to tell their friends and family about their surgery, because family get-togethers are very important in our society. Ultimately, the responsibility is yours, but you'll be much more successful in the long run if everyone's on the same page and tries to help you achieve your goals.

"I'll Be Good Tomorrow" Doesn't Work

Don't fool yourself into thinking that consuming fewer calories the day after a holiday or the week after vacation will work. An excessive dinner or party can undo a lot of treadmill walking. I recommend planning in advance and exercising a little every day for an entire week before the party. Don't try telling yourself that you'll make up for your indulgences the day after the party, unless you can safely commit to six hours at the gym! If you're going on a cruise, sign up for an activity that gets you walking or exercising every day. Nearly every boat and hotel has a gym, physical outings, or a map of local walking trails these days. Keep in mind that walking one mile burns 100 calories for 130 pounds of body weight. If you weigh 260 pounds, you will burn 200 calories for each mile you walk. That means you'll have to walk three miles to burn off just one margarita! Because margaritas usually come with chips and dip, expect to need another three-mile walk. And if you add fried ice cream and churros for dessert, add a third walk. Walking nine miles takes a lot of time, but consuming those treats takes just a few minutes. That's why a full week of extra exercise is needed to make up for one evening of decadence.

Beware of the Booze

Besides containing a lot of empty calories, alcoholic beverages lower your inhibitions, making you more likely to choose poor food options. Drinks are also often served with high-calorie snacks, like trail mix or beer nuts. These calories add up. Do not think that forgoing a nutritious dinner will cancel out the calories in a frozen daiquiri, either. If you're hungry when you start drinking, you will be far more likely to eat high-fat and high-calorie foods.

Allow Yourself a Taste of Your "Favorite"

Did you know that the chemical triggers that evoke our desires for a certain food are satisfied within the first two or three bites? So, if key lime pie is your favorite (like it is for one of my patients), then allow yourself just two or three bites. Understand the choice you are making and leave the guilt at home, but stick to just a small taste (each bite may contain 50 calories or more). Since it may be hard to push away the rest of the slice, make sure your initial portion is quite small. Then you can safely clean your plate! Or share one dessert with three friends. If you allow yourself these tastes from time to time, you'll be less likely to overdo it when you're confronted with your favorite food.

Think about Feeling Full

It takes 20 to 25 minutes from the time you eat until chemical and stretch receptors in your stomach send the message to your brain to signal satiety. So, don't wolf down your food like it's a race to the finish. Instead, slow down. Taste your food, enjoy your company, and approach your mealtime like a leisurely Sunday drive through the countryside. A good trick is to make sure to put your fork down between every bite. If you do this, not only will you learn to recognize when you're full, it will probably take you longer than others to get through your meal so you won't have time for a second helping.

In addition to the above, the following are good reminders for gastric sleeve patients.

Remember the First Rule

What is the First Rule of WLS Eating? Protein First! That means pass on the chips and dips, appetizers, finger foods, etc., and focus on good protein, like fish, tofu, beans, chicken, or turkey. Once you have eaten your protein, then you can have a vegetable side dish (remember the Second Rule?).

No WLS Likes a Sloppy Drunk

Excessive alcohol intake is one of the worst enemies of social eating for WLS patients. Besides the extra calories, the loss of inhibition will make it harder to listen to your pressure signals that you've had enough. It's also less likely that you'll remember to take small bites and chew your food well. This could lead to a very embarrassing social situation. Eat your protein first, wait 30 minutes, then consume an alcoholic beverage, if you choose. But make sure to plan your alcohol consumption carefully to avoid taking in too many extra calories.

A complex salad is a Good Choice; an iceberg lettuce salad is not

Despite its reputation as a health food, the typical appetizer salad that accompanies a meal at a restaurant is often low in nutrition and lacking in true flavor. This usually leads to a dependency on dressings to make it palatable, and many salad dressings are dense in calories and fat. Choose a large complex salad as your main entrée. The more colors, the better. Load it full of fresh veggies for intense flavor (remember the Third Rule?). Top it with a lean protein for a complete meal!

Enjoy the holidays or vacation, focus on friends and family, fit in some time for walking or other exercise—or better yet, make time for active "play"—and make smart food choices whenever you can!

The 21 Days Exception

Many New Year's resolutions are about exercising and dieting. Eager people seek out local gyms and sign up for memberships with the intention of really changing their lives. But how long do you think these good intentions generally last? Most New Year's resolutions are broken within 21 days. Then these hopefuls go back to their old ways for the remaining 344 days of the year. Of course, there are always some who are able to make it a couple of months, and a rare few who stick with it maybe even several months. But eventually, the little things of daily life get in the way—the late meeting at work, the child's ballet class, the sick parent, the car that breaks down, the vacation planning, etc. Some will make a good effort to get back on track, and there may be a slight renewal of dedication to the gym, but usually by summer and all of the trips and camps, you're off track again. Does this sound familiar?

I tell my patients that we have it backwards. Instead of "sticking to it" for 21 days, then being bad the other 344 days, my patients strive to be good for most of the year and pick 21 occasions to celebrate. I call this

THE 21 DAYS EXCEPTION.

I typically try not to assign terms like "good", "bad", "treat", and "splurge" to describe healthy living. (I have consciously used these words in a few situations in this book, however, to reflect the accepted attitudes of many frustrated dieters.) Lifestyle is really a matter of choices we all have to make on a daily basis. If I choose to have a big salad for lunch every day at work, then that is my norm. I'm not on a "diet", nor am I "trying to be healthy". It's just me being me. This is what I try to teach my patients. So, when I choose to deviate from this norm, then I know it's just a choice I've made. I'm not "splurging". I'm definitely not "treating myself". I've already been treating myself well with vitality, strength, and stamina from eating those salads!

During group, when we go around in a circle trying to name 21 special occasions, everyone gets the easy ones first—Thanksgiving, Christmas, wedding anniversary, Valentine's, birthdays, etc. Then we start to stall a little. Pushing my patients harder, they usually come up with Mother's Day, Father's Day, a child's wedding, Fourth of July, Halloween. Then people start reaching for answers—seven-day cruise, Labor Day cookout, family reunion. Someone who's Irish might say St. Patrick's Day. Someone who is Jewish might name all eight days of Chanukah. Someone who comes from a big family might want to celebrate all five kids' birthdays. Yet, we seldom reach 21! So you see, it is possible to be healthy and not feel like you're missing out on the special occasions. What are YOUR 21 special days? Name those special occasions that add an extra dose of happiness to your life. Understand that they are special in ways that may be personal, so the answers you give might be very different from those of your loved ones.

---

344 IS FAR GREATER THAN 21.

It's the patterns established over 344 days—and not the deviance from that pattern on 21 days—that will influence your overall health.

Final Thoughts

Although you've reached the end of this book, you have certainly not reached the end of the road. My hope is that this book has demonstrated that you can reach your goals and, more importantly, that you can always set new ones. I know a lot has changed in my life since the writing of my last book, and I am guessing a lot has changed for you recently as well. My hopes are that most of the changes have been for the better. Leading and maintaining a healthy lifestyle is an ongoing process, and there is always room for improvement. We all experience setbacks. We all have challenges. But isn't it nice to know that, on any day, if you are not happy with where you are in your life, you can choose to change it? The key is that you keep doing small things on a daily basis that will eventually add up to big results.

One of the most effective ways to keep on track is to continually educate yourself on the many facets of health. Now that you've finished this book, perhaps you might be interested in researching food safety, walking programs, local volunteering activities, childhood nutrition, personal development, the "grow local" movement, or anything else that has piqued your interest.

As you continue on your journey, keep the following tips in mind. Over time, they will become automatic habits:

- **Remember the Three Rules.** They provide you with a strong understanding for all of your food choices. Many health tips you read about stem from the Three Rules, for example:

    o **Eat like a caveman**—This means you should avoid processed and pre-packaged foods. Eat fresh, cook your own meals, and fill your plate with mostly non-animal protein and vegetables. Despite our preconceived notions, cavemen didn't actually eat much meat because it was not readily available and was difficult to obtain (hunting was dangerous and exhausting). They were mostly gatherers.

    o **Eat a variety of color**—When you look at the typical plate of an overweight person—a plate that is loaded with chicken-fried steak, mashed potatoes and gravy, and a dinner roll for example—you will notice the predominance of one color: yellow in various shades, like beige or tan. In other words, the color of FAT. Isn't it ironic that while many people struggle with their weight, the food they eat is the color of the substance they are trying to avoid? You can easily correct this. Start by adding one item of food that has a different color, like broccoli, and then go from there. But don't fool yourself. If you cover your broccoli with cheese sauce, you've just turned your green food back into (you guessed it) yellow goo! You can never go wrong by adding more leafy greens to any dish. Eating a variety of colors is also a good way to ensure that you are getting better nutrition and consuming fewer calories, because you will be eating more fresh produce.

o **Avoid the white carbs**—Steer clear of foods made with processed white flour like white bread, white pasta, chips, crackers, and all of the "little restaurant extras."

- **Exercise a little every day.** Remember, if you break one bead of sweat, it counts as exercise. Whenever you can, aim to do more continuous exercise of a higher intensity. But if you don't have a free hour to devote to exercise some days, spend ten or fifteen minutes moving around anyway. Remember, the patterns you establish add up!

- **Give up on diets**—Why "**Die**-it" when you can "**Live**-it"? Where has dieting gotten you all of these years? It's time to do something different. Start by rethinking your self-worth. Understand what a valuable person you are and recognize that you deserve a better life! How much has the world missed out on because you are not participating fully in life? It's time for you to get back out there and Live It! A diet is a short-term, quick fix that will ultimately fail you; instead, ensure you are taking proactive steps to live the life you want.

- **Be happy**—My goal for patients is to have them love food again, love themselves, and take pride in their accomplishments. If you slip up, take stock of all you have accomplished and set reasonable goals for what you can do today (e.g., a 20-minute lunchtime walk? A home-cooked dinner? Healthy lunch choices?). It's all the little choices we make hundreds of times each day that determine whether or not we will succeed. **344 is much greater than 21.**

Think about how what you consume makes you feel. I know this sounds all New Age Touchy-Feely and such, but it has real merit. You have to understand what role food plays in your life, how comforting it is, why it helps you to relax, what pain it is relieving, and what issue it covers up that you are not wanting to face. This is often the most frightening step to becoming healthier—baring your soul so that you can examine it, for all of its faults, but also for all of its wonders! Then seek more effective ways to feel better and relax that won't sabotage your health. Reach out to friends, enjoy evening walks, and find other strategies to get the emotional benefits you may have been looking for in food. If you find Happiness, chances are you will also find Thinness and Wellness.

- **Take time every day to make yourself better**—At the end of every cartoon, G.I.Joe says, "Now you know, and KNOWING is half the battle!" It is crucial to become more informed about nutrition. Just be sure to seek real information, not fad diets, scams, or cheats. Find a well-researched book by someone with solid credentials. Don't rely on the materials in the checkout aisle of the grocery store, but instead try books like *Fast Food Nation* by Eric Schlosser or *What to Eat* by Marion Nestle. You can also learn new skills: gardening, cooking, meditation, handling stress, you name it! I'm sure you will find a video about almost anything you could want to learn on YouTube.

- **Write down your goals**—Thomas Jefferson once said, "If you want something you've never had, you must be willing to do something you've never done." This is the key to success in any and all endeavors, not just weight loss. Your goals and desires take on a whole new life and meaning when you commit them to paper. When writing your goals, be specific ("I will walk for 30 minutes 3 days per week," instead of "I will exercise") and be true to who you are (if you hate going to the gym, do not waste money on a new gym membership.) If you want a life worth living, then you must set BIG GOALS that are worth reaching and be willing to commit them to paper.

While in pursuit of your goals, make small changes that add up. For example, you might think it is silly to write a lofty goal like "I want to win the Boston Marathon" when you don't even own a pair of running shoes. But I say,

> *"Do it! Go for that big goal."*

Just start with small steps. It's the small changes we can stick to that are sustainable over the long haul, and that will eventually add up to the big change in your health. Once your small changes become second nature, add another and then another. Do this throughout the year, and you'll have adopted a much healthier lifestyle without having to overhaul your entire existence. So, start small and build up momentum to reach your big goals. And if you don't win the Boston marathon, maybe you'll still run it!

- **Remember that you are worth it.** Focus on surrounding yourself with positive reinforcement and people who want to help you succeed. Positive reinforcement starts with the quiet, little stories you tell yourself in your head every day. Stories are made up of words. So to change these stories, you have to change the words you use.

Remember this illustration?

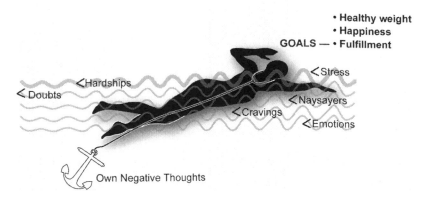

When you first saw it, you probably thought, "How will I ever lose that anchor around my neck?" Here's how:

CHANGE THE WORDS YOU USE

Words to Avoid	Words to Use
TRY, "I will try."	DO, "I will do."
HARD, "That's hard to do."	EASY, "Running is easy."
AM NOT, "I am not a good cook."	AM, "I am a good learner."
CAN'T, "I can't do it."	CAN, "I can start a garden."
WISH, "I wish my spouse would..."	PLAN, "We plan together."
HOPE, "I hope it gets better."	MAKE, "I make it so."
IF ONLY, "If only ___would change."	MUST, "I must change."
SOMEDAY, "Someday, I'll..."	NOW, "Why not now?"

Stop saying things like "I'm trying to lose weight." What's the first thing you do after you realize you've lost something? You try to find it! Is it any surprise that your weight has yo-yo'ed all these years? After losing the weight, you start looking for it, and guess what? You find it...plus some! So instead, say,

> *"I'm making my health and happiness a priority."*

Your health is vital and should never take a backseat to all your other obligations. And your happiness never depends on the actions of others. Stop "trying" and start "doing." Pretend you are the swimmer in the illustration and write in your own goals. Go participate in life and show the WORLD that you are WORTH it!

Remember to come back and review your answers in this book every few months. They will help you gauge how far you've come. You might also want to join a local support group or start your own, using this book as your guide. You can also send me a note or write on my Facebook wall. Just search for "Duc Vuong" and then add me as a friend. Remember, the answer lies within you. Now go out and make a difference in the world.

www.ultimategastricsleeve.com

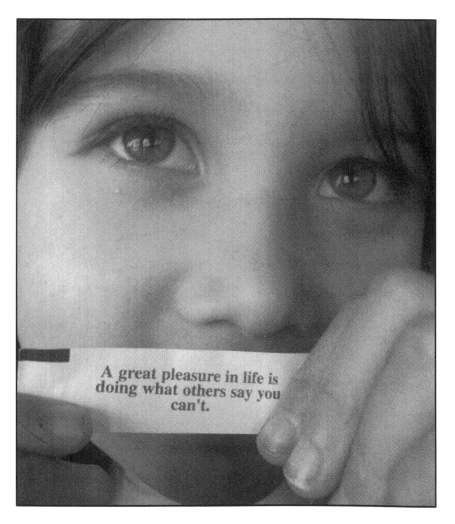

A great pleasure in life is doing what others say you can't.

--Kizzie Vuong, Age 6

Appendix A: The Three Rules

Rule #1: Protein first.

- Not "Protein only"
- Not "Protein mostly"
- Not "Protein always"

Rule #2: Fill your pouch with the most nutritious food you can, most of the time.

- "Fill your pouch" — Protein first, because protein keeps you full longer

- "With the most nutritious food you can" — Protein first, because if you are eating some sort of protein first, then I know you are getting some sort of nutrition.

- "Most of the time" — Because life happens. It is what you do most of the time on an everyday basis that will determine how successful you are in weight loss and in life.

Rule #3 (Kizzie's Rule): You can eat all of the fresh fruits and vegetables you want, any time you want, as much as you want.

- Because pound for pound, fresh fruits and vegetables are the most nutritious foods.
- Because no one has ever said, "I'm overweight because I eat too many fruits and vegetables."
- This rule applies even if you are a diabetic.
- Canned fruits and vegetables do not count. They must be fresh!

Appendix B: The Texture Scale™

Typically: Typically:
Lower Nutritional Value   Higher Calories
Lower Fat   Higher Fat
                    ←---IDEAL RANGE-----------------→

1_____2_____3_____4_____5_____6___

Water   Mushy Foods   Fish   Shrimp/Seafood   Chicken   Steak
        Shakes   Fresh Fruits/Veggies   Dark White
        Boiled Veggies Tofu/Egg Whites   Turkey   P o r k

- No limit on Water
- No bread on the scale
- No sodas
- No category labeled "junk"
- Chips are a "liquid"
- Scale can be dynamic, depending on how the food item is prepared
- Reheated foods are typically thicker than when initially prepared
- Eat between Textures 3-4 MOST of the time, with occasional forays into 5-6
- If you lived your whole life and never ate red meat again, you'd be happier and healthier!

Appendix C: Mushy Food Syndrome

Typically: Typically:

Lower Nutritional Value   Higher Calories

Lower Fat   Higher Fat

←---IDEAL RANGE-----------------→

1	2	3	4	5	6
Water	Mushy Foods	Fish	Shrimp/Seafood	Chicken	Steak
	Shakes	Fresh Fruits/Veggies		Dark White	
	Boiled Veggies	Tofu/Egg Whites		Turkey	P o r k

Mushy foods—also known as slider foods—are Texture Scale #2, such as mashed potatoes, refried beans, and pudding. These foods are typically higher in calories and lower in nutrients.

What will happen to your weight if you eat foods that are relatively higher in calories?

Weight loss plateau or you will regain weight.

What will your energy be like if you regularly eat foods that are typically low in nutrition?

Low energy level

What will your attitude be like if you have no energy?

Poor or bad attitude, frustrated

"Dr. Vuong, I have no energy, I am barely eating, and gosh, darn it—I'm not even losing weight!" = Mushy Food Syndrome

Appendix D: Protein Sources

Again, this is probably the area of greatest departure for me from my previous books. It is important that we, as an entire society, start consuming more natural, non-animal-based sources of protein. I cannot emphasize that enough. This list is not intended to be complete, but rather to serve as an idea generator and reminder for you. Buy organic and locally-grown whenever possible.

BEST—EAT THESE DAILY

- Vegetables—like broccoli

- Beans—green, lima, pinto, etc. as well as lentils

- Soy Products—tofu, edamame, soy milk

- Whole Grains—couscous, bulgar, and quinoa

- Nuts—almonds, walnuts; not peanut butter

- Fish—fresh, preferably wild-caught, and definitely not from a can.

ACCEPTABLE OCCASIONALLY

- Chicken—even skinless chicken should be eaten only on occasion

- Turkey—not much better than chicken

SAVE FOR SPECIAL OCCASIONS ONLY

- Meat—beef is too high in fat. Don't be fooled by "It's a lean cut of meat." Maybe it's "leaner" compared to other cuts of meat, but it is still too high in fat.

- Pork is also a red meat. Game meat is better, but can still be high in fat.

- Dairy

- o   No one should drink whole milk on a daily basis, except for baby cows.

- o   Choose artisan cheeses, and use them sparingly.

- o   No "processed cheese products"

- Protein Supplements—for convenience, but not to rely on regularly

Works Cited

Caffeine Questions: How Much is Too Much? abcnews.go.com, 23 October, 2012.

Centers for Disease Control and Prevention. Division of Nutrition and Physical Activity. *Research to Practice Series No. 2: Portion Size*. Atlanta: 2006. Print.

Gehrer, S et al. "Fewer Nutrient Deficiencies After Laparscopic Sleeve Gastrectomy (LSG) than After Laparoscopic Roux-Y-Gastric Bypass (LRYGB)—a Prospective Study." *Obes. Surg.* (2010) 20:447-453.

Oliveira AB, et al. "The Impact of Organic Farming on Quality of Tomatoes Is Associated to Increased Oxidative Stress during Fruit Development." *PLoS ONE* 8.2 (2013): e56354. doi:10.1371/journal.pone.0056354. Web.

Pilzer, PZ. *The New Wellness Revolution: How to Make a Fortune in the Next Trillion Dollar Industry, 2nd ed.* Hoboken: John Wiley 7Sons, Inc. 2007.

Snyder-Marlow, G., et al. "Nutrition Care for Patients Undergoing Laparoscopic Sleeve Gastrectomy for Weight Loss." *J AM DIET ASSOC.* (2010) 110:600-607.

Wiley AS. "Milk Intake and Total Dairy Consumption: Associations with Early Menarche in NHANES 1999-2004." *PLoS ONE* 6.2 (2011): e14685. doi:10.1371/journal.pone.0014685. Web.

Made in the USA
San Bernardino, CA
22 June 2018